A Colour Atlas of
Forensic Dentistry

A Colour Atlas of
FORENSIC DENTISTRY

D.K. Whittaker
BDS, Ph.D, FDSRCS, Dip.F.Od.(LHMC)
Reader in Oral Biology,
University of Wales College of Medicine
Consultant Dental Surgeon

D.G. MacDonald
RD[*], BDS, Ph.D, FRC Path, FDSRCPS(G)
Reader in Oral Medicine and Pathology,
University of Glasgow
Consultant Oral Pathologist

Wolfe Medical Publications Ltd

Copyright © D. K. Whittaker and D. G. MacDonald, 1989
Published by Wolfe Publishing Ltd, 1989
Printed by W.S. Cowell Ltd, Ipswich, England
ISBN 0 7234 0961 7

A CIP catalogue record for this book is available from the
British Library.

This book is one of the titles in the series of Wolfe Medical
Atlases, a series that brings together the world's largest
systematic published collection of diagnostic colour
photographs.

For a full list of Atlases in the series, plus forthcoming titles
and details of our surgical, dental and veterinary Atlases,
please write to Wolfe Medical Publications Ltd, 2-16
Torrington Place, London WC1E 7LT, England.

Contents

Preface

We have been encouraged to write this book by colleagues in the dental profession who from time to time are requested to provide information to the police concerning their patients, and also by friends and colleagues in many disciplines who collaborate towards a common goal, the pursuit of justice. The authors are experienced practitioners of forensic dentistry who have been closely associated with the development of the subject over the past two decades, and who lecture widely to professional groups both within and outside their own profession.

Although forensic dentistry has close links with its parent discipline, forensic medicine, it is concerned not so much with the cause of injury or death, but with identification of the victim. There is, however, a degree of overlap, in that the teeth may be used as weapons against a victim by an assailant or as a defence by a victim against an attacker.

It is the role of the forensic dentist to offer advice and opinion to the courts in matters lying within his professional training and experience, and he or she usually does this on invitation from the investigators involved in a case. These may be the forensic pathologist, the coroner or other appropriate legal authority, the lawyer, the police or the forensic scientist. In the UK the forensic dentist has no official status over and above his or her professional position as a qualified dental surgeon, and indeed the courts may seek advice from any dentist whom they feel to be most able to provide it. The collection of dental evidence, its interpretation and its presentation in a form most useful to those requesting it, may be judged to be most adequately realized by individuals who have made a special study of the particular techniques involved, and there is an increasing tendency to rely on a relatively few specialists who have so prepared themselves. At present there is little or no formal training in this sphere of activity, and forensic dentists may be drawn from hospital consultants, academics or general practitioners.

Theoretically, any dental advice sought by the courts would fall within a broad definition of forensic dentistry but, by custom, legal reports on injuries to living patients, opinions on the prognosis of such injuries and the likelihood of further treatment would usually be sought either from the practitioner directly concerned with the care of the patient or from a consultant to whom the patient or the dental records may be referred. The generally accepted realm of forensic dentistry or odontology is therefore commonly restricted to matters normally outside the experience of clinical practice and involving criminal activity—sudden death, injuries to third parties caused by the teeth, and identification of specimens or unknown bodies by reference to the dentition and previous dental records.

It may be considered that the best preparation for such activity is a sound understanding of the principles of general dental surgery, and a particular interest in the development, growth and age changes in the teeth, the supporting structures and the facial bones and soft tissues. Added to this must be experience in the application of this knowledge and specialized laboratory techniques to the legal situation. Finally, the forensic dentist must be prepared to present his dental findings in a manner most likely to be helpful to those who are charged with prosecuting the due purposes of the law.

There have been a number of excellent texts covering particular specialized aspects of forensic dentistry, and in the main these have been written for the forensic odontologist. They have therefore sought to include, with varying degrees of success, not only the principles of basic dental science upon which the subject is based, but also examples of the manner in which this information may be applied in particular cases. This scientific basis is more properly dealt with in specialized texts of oral embryology, development, anatomy and histology, supplemented by texts in clinical dental surgery, and it would be a magnum opus which sought to cover these aspects in the detail required by the specialist in addition to describing the application of this information in particular investigations.

It is not our intention in this small volume to provide a comprehensive text for the specialist, nor indeed to attempt to examine exhaustively all the problems which the practising forensic dentist might encounter, but rather to review the general principles involved. We are aware that in situations requiring the peculiar expertise of the forensic dentist many other professionals are involved at various stages of the investigation, and cooperation can be most productive when all are aware of the scope and limitations of each other's contributions. Our approach has been to provide as much information as possible in a form acceptable to a broad readership. We have eschewed jargon and specialist terminology in favour of a visual form of presentation. It is our hope that the illustrations contained in this Atlas, supplemented by no more than the minimum necessary text, will meet the needs of undergraduate and postgraduate dentists and our colleagues in forensic medicine, forensic science, the police and the legal profession who require a handy reference manual to the basic principles of our craft. Forensic dentists, we believe, have much to offer in the pursuit of justice and if this book does no more than suggest useful avenues of investigation to our colleagues it will achieve our main objective.

D.K. Whittaker
D.G. MacDonald

Acknowledgements

Most of the illustrations have been prepared from our own cases. We are particularly grateful to Frank Hartles, Head of the Dental Illustration Unit in Cardiff and in Glasgow to Michael Broad, Instructor in Dental Technology, and the staff of the Dental Illustration Unit.

Special thanks are due to our clinical colleagues for permission to use slides of their cases, to the photographic units of the several police forces with whom we have worked, and also to the following people and organizations: illustration 8 Wiltshire Police; 139 G. Webster; 209 to 213 P. Coleman; 214 to 217, 220 to 221, 223 to 231 D.H. Clark and Kenyon Emergency Services; 218 to 219 and 222 West Yorkshire Police; 269, 277, 281 and 285 British Museum (Natural History).

Suzy Read, Pauline Ballett, Alexandra Garven and Jessie Davis have patiently typed and retyped the manuscript. If there are any errors, they are ours.

Chapter 1
The scope of forensic dentistry

The forensic dentist is usually invited to assist in a particular investigation by the police, the forensic services or a forensic pathologist. In most cases the problem will be one of identification of an unknown corpse, and it is important that examination is systematic so that no information is missed.

The purpose of this Atlas is to describe procedures leading to a positive identification, but in many instances exclusion of an individual from the case may be a useful part of the investigation.

This introductory chapter is intended to provide a brief overview of some of the problems which may be encountered, and to indicate the type of situation in which the forensic dentist could be expected to offer useful advice and opinion. The dentist is rarely, if ever, the first expert to be called, and there is evidence to suggest that in a substantial number of investigations a dentist is not invited to participate because no-one has recognized that there were any dental implications in the case.

The applications of forensic dentistry are expanding as the science develops. In addition to identification procedures of whole or fragmented bodies, the dentist may help with problems involving ageing, racial origins, habits and occupations, previous dental history and procedures, the study of fragments of jaws and teeth and the soft tissues of the mouth. Information can be gained from dentures and from bite marks, the comparison of dental records, liaison with members of the dental profession, and in mass disasters. This is not an exhaustive list but is intended to suggest to the non-dental investigator grounds for seeking advice in this specialized area.

The teeth may be as unique as a fingerprint, but it is more difficult to provide from teeth identification evidence that will be acceptable to the courts. It is the extraction, cataloguing and interpretation of tooth data which form a large part of the science of forensic odontology. In most instances there is no ideal or proven technique, and flexibility, an open mind and a willingness to learn are necessary attributes of the dentist involved in this type of work.

Non-dental identification

Simpler methods of identification are always attempted before the forensic dentist is approached: in most cases, these are successful.

Most recently dead individuals are identified by facial recognition by a relative or acquaintance. Identification is by nuances of facial shape and colour which may be difficult to describe, and there is usually relatively little change in the countenance in the early stages following death (Chapter 2).

Disfiguration may follow trauma, burning or putrefaction, when it would not be appropriate to ask the next-of-kin to examine the body. If facial features cannot be used, then in a few cases a fingerprint may be taken, even from bodies which have undergone advanced decomposition. If a similar print is on police record, or some indication of the identity of the individual is known allowing fingerprints to be taken from household surroundings, a positive identification may be possible. Modern techniques enable fingerprints to be 'lifted' from materials which previously would not have yielded a clear image, and comparison with prints on record may now be possible using computerized pattern recognition.

Identification from teeth

There remain a few cases where neither of these methods can satisfactorily be used. Hands and fingers may be mutilated or damaged following putrefaction, fire or prolonged immersion in water. Under most conditions occurring in nature the teeth are the least destructible part of the body and they may readily survive all of these changes. Not only is there a wealth of naturally acquired information within these teeth, but changes brought about by age or pathology, or by the intervention of the dental surgeon, result in the mouth becoming unique to the individual and providing a library from which information may be extracted at any time and for considerable periods after death. This information may on occasions be difficult of access, and specialized techniques are required (Chapter 3).

Occasionally the features of an individual may be well preserved, but there may be no clue as to identity and therefore no means of approaching possible relatives. The information contained within the dental structures may be used to build a dossier of the age, social habits, racial origin, dental history and peculiarities of the individual. This may eventually enable a positive identification to be made. Examinations in this field must be carried out by experienced dental surgeons who have a broad training both in basic dental science and in clinical dentistry.

Most parts of the body undergo changes as an individual ages and are gradually or rapidly replaced or cycled, depending upon the type of tissue involved. The teeth, and particularly the enamel, are unique in that once physiological or growth information is built into them they may remain stable for thousands of years after death (Chapter 4). Individuals who have been subjected to extensive restorative procedures such as metallic fillings may unwittingly be carrying their visiting card in their oral cavity. The purpose of fillings, crowns and complex bridges is to restore the shape and functional activity of the individual teeth following trauma, wear or the ravages of decay. Each restoration is unique to that individual. The variety of materials which may be used, the manner in which they are placed, the skill of the workmanship and the changes in the teeth following their insertion may be indicators not only of the identity of the individual in whom they are found, but may say something about the dentist or dentists who had worked in that particular mouth (Chapter 5).

An examination of the teeth may occasionally provide a clue as to the racial origin of an individual, or, if unusual dentistry is present, to the racial origin of the dentist.

Certain occupations may also leave their marks on the teeth. Carpenters holding nails between the incisal edges of the anterior teeth or hairdressers holding hairclips may eventually produce notched defects which the forensic dentist may relate to a particular occupation. It is, for example, well recognized that frequent playing of certain brass or wind instruments may produce permanent changes in the dentition and information of this nature may help to solve an otherwise difficult case. In recent times occupational health inspectors and dental surgeons have become more aware of these problems and improvements in occupational environment and habits mean that these markers are becoming increasingly rare.

Information from a study of skull bones

In the case of an unborn fetus, a young child, an adolescent or a young adult it may be possible to determine the age at death with reasonable accuracy from a study of the bones of the skull. In older people this becomes more difficult. Although at first sight this may not be judged to be within the scope of forensic dentistry, in fact dentists are trained to study the whole skull in relation to growth and disease processes in the structures supporting and surrounding the teeth and oral cavity.

Other useful information which may be obtained from studies of skull bones is the determination of sex and racial origin, and perhaps of positive identification (Chapter 6).

By examination of the healing of an extraction socket it may be possible to determine the time since extraction of a tooth. The bone of the skeleton is more susceptible to changes induced by its environment than are the teeth, but both structures may absorb minerals from the soil in which they were buried or may release minerals into the surrounding environment. The protein matrix of bone changes slowly after death and attempts have been made to determine the time of death from chemical changes occurring in the skeleton. These estimations are not precise but, taken in conjunction with conditions at the scene of burial, may allow an opinion as to the length of time elapsed since death.

Oral tissues and fluids

In general, the soft tissues are not so useful as the hard tissues in forensic investigations because putrefaction or damage by other means may destroy information. Positive identification may occasionally be achieved from intra-oral tattoos. Tattooing of this nature is a rather painful and uncommon event and it may be assumed that people would subject themselves to such a procedure only if the tattoo was of some particular significance.

Pigmentation of the lining of the mouth, the presence of disease, or changes caused by the ingestion of certain drugs may help to differentiate one individual from another (Chapter 7) but it has to be admitted that in most cases the soft tissues provide much less information than the teeth and bones.

Although little use has been made of the individuality of 'lip' patterns in the United Kingdom, this aspect of identification procedures has been studied for some years in Japan. It may be that more detailed studies of the lines and grooves on the lips may pay dividends, but the number of cases in which a 'print' of the lips may be left at the scene of a crime will necessarily be small.

Ageing the dead from the teeth

The teeth not only provide information as to the dental history of an individual, and perhaps a hint as to his or her origins or habits, but because teeth develop chronologically, their degree of development or eruption in the mouth cavity at any given time enables an approximation of the age of the individual to be calculated.

Age determination may still be possible even in older people when the teeth have completed development and are relatively stable in the mouth. Certain changes occur within the tooth which enable an age estimation of the older unknown body to be made. For example, translucency of the root apex increases with age and so a determination of its extent can provide information as to the age of the owner of the tooth (Chapter 8).

The older a person becomes, the more inaccurate will be an age determination from the teeth but, in practice, the techniques illustrated in this Atlas often prove to be the most successful method of ageing skeletal material when one or more teeth are present.

Dentures

Identification of a body is made more difficult if some or all of the teeth are missing, a situation which is all too commonly found in older age groups. Cast metal dentures are individually designed either by the dentist or the dental technician and the nuances of design and manufacture may be useful in an identification procedure. A more difficult problem is presented by the all-acrylic denture, which usually conforms to a standard design and has no significantly unique features to aid in identification of the wearer. Fortunately, some dentures are marked and can be traced to a particular owner, but it is essential in such cases to demonstrate that the denture had been worn by the victim and was not discarded at the scene by someone else (Chapters 9 and 10).

The material from which a denture has been made sometimes helps in identification, and the type of teeth fitted to the denture and the standard of workmanship may also be useful pointers.

If a denture is found at the scene of a crime a mould or cast of the jaw which it fitted may be prepared and finally compared to the jaw of a suspect. Although not nearly so useful in forensic investigations as the natural teeth, there are many ways in which information may be acquired from a set of false teeth.

Laboratory procedures

Small fragments of tooth material are sometimes discovered at the scene of a crime or in other suspicious circumstances. If a number of fragments or individual teeth are found it may be possible to determine the number of people from whom the teeth were evulsed. Biochemical changes in teeth and bones after death may indicate that an attempt has been made to dispose of certain parts of the body, but they may also be caused naturally by chemicals found in the locality where the body was deposited. It may be necessary to take soil and water samples from the scene at which the body was found. In one case barnacles adhering to the surface of a skull, which was buried some distance from the nearest coast, indicated that the skull must have been transferred there from a marine environment.

Soft tissues, tissue fluids and fragments of the bones of the jaws may yield useful information. The permission of the coroner must always be sought before specimens are removed for laboratory examination, and less destructive techniques such as radiographs, impressions and study models, and a careful examination of the parts in situ should always precede removal of teeth or the jaws themselves. Excised specimens may be examined in a more leisurely and careful manner than is possible in the intact mouth,

and there is the added advantage that they can be permanently preserved.

Some areas of investigation fall outside the immediate expertise of clinical dentistry but are important forensically. An example of such a technique is the extraction of proteins from the fluids and living processes in the dentine of a fragment of tooth left at the scene of a crime. These proteins contain information about the blood group or enzyme groups of the individual from whom the tooth fragment came and may help to eliminate a suspect if not positively confirm association with a crime (Chapter 11).

Dental and medical records

All the information from an unknown body is of little value unless ante-mortem dental records can be acquired with which to compare the post-mortem data. This comparison should always be done by an expert trained in forensic techniques as allowances often have to be made for incorrect or incomplete records which, in themselves, may not necessarily rule out a satisfactory identification.

Ante-mortem records may take the form of photographs showing characteristics of the teeth, descriptions by relatives of the teeth or of missing or fractured teeth. Additionally, there may be professional records such as written dental charts, radiographs, impressions, study casts, clinical photographs of particular dental conditions or restorations fitted in the mouth. It is important that the information collected by the forensic dentist from the mouth of an unknown body be catalogued and described before reference is made to ante-mortem records. In this way the examiner is unbiased and does not consciously or subconsciously adapt the findings. Any differences between the post-mortem and ante-mortem records must be satisfactorily explained or no identification can be assumed (Chapter 12).

Occasionally, the expertise of the forensic dentist may be useful in areas of the body distant from the oral cavity. Foreign objects, such as parts of dental appliances or instruments, may occasionally be inhaled into the lungs from the oral cavity via the larynx. Ante-mortem medical records may then enable comparisons to be made with the features seen in a body requiring identification.

The mass disaster

The methods described in this Atlas are most frequently applied to cases involving only one or a few individuals. If identifications are required in disasters where a large number of people is involved, the same, or similar techniques may be applied but in addition there are considerable problems of an organizational nature which need to be attended to (Chapter 13).

In some mass disasters, such as air crashes where fragmentation of bodies often occurs, dental forensic techniques may help to identify personnel in as many as 70 per cent of cases. Special training, preparation and experience are a great advantage in mass disasters as time is often at a premium and the workload may be huge.

Bite mark analysis

The burden of activity of the forensic dentist is directed towards identification of the unknown dead using the techniques already outlined, but a significant and additional proportion of the dentist's work may be to advise on the likelihood of a particular assailant having attacked a victim using his teeth as a weapon.

Bite mark comparisons are particularly important in cases with sexual overtones and also in cases of non-accidental injury to children. In the latter case it may be important for the forensic dentist to distinguish between a bite on a child produced by a brother or sister, or a bite produced by a parent or relative accused of assault. The analysis of bite marks both on the living and the dead requires considerable experience, as there are many pitfalls in associating a particular mark with a particular dentition (Chapter 14).

Bites may on occasions be left in foodstuff or other objects found at the scene of a crime and it may be possible to match the teeth of a suspect to these marks (Chapter 15) or, equally importantly, to eliminate a suspect from an enquiry.

Archaeological finds

Not all human remains found under unusual circumstances are of direct interest to the law enforcement agencies. Human skeletal material and teeth withstand the passage of time remarkably well, thereby allowing us to study not only Egyptian civilizations living around 5,000 years ago but even fossil man separated from us by more than two million years.

Forensic dentistry can aid the anthropologist, the palaeopathologist and the archaeologist in their study of early man, but can also advise contemporary interested parties that they are dealing with cases that will never come to trial because the perpetrators will have died decades or centuries ago (Chapter 16).

Chapter 2
Equipment and examination of the body

The forensic dentist is usually invited to examine a body or portions of a body by the police or by the Home Office pathologist or forensic services. The complexities may not be apparent at initial examination, and as there is no way of predicting the outcome every effort should be made to be as comprehensive as possible, even though the case may be solved via some other route and the dental evidence becomes unimportant.

A great deal of information may be acquired using simple techniques of observation without the need to damage or destroy the specimens. This approach should always be used initially before resorting to a full post-mortem examination and before specialized laboratory techniques are brought into use.

Usually the remains will already have been moved to a convenient mortuary before the forensic dentist is called, so the standard instruments will be available. Any additional equipment should be provided by the visiting dentist, and it is essential that a specialized examination kit is available at all times in a readily transportable form. Inevitably, personal preferences develop for certain items and therefore only those which are generally agreed to be necessary will be described. In the absence of particular difficulties, the forensic dentist examines the body in the same sequence in which a living patient would be examined. First the extra-oral condition of the body is assessed, followed by an intra-oral clinical examination, supplemented where necessary by appropriate radiographs.

The foregoing comments apply to most cases in which the forensic dentist is involved —notably identification procedures. Different requirements apply to bite mark cases and these are detailed in Chapters 14 and 15.

The scene of the incident

1 Collecting the evidence. It is unusual for the dentist to be called directly to the scene of a crime, but this may occur where dental evidence is obviously important. The team will have isolated the site and the position of the body and any other specimens will have been recorded by photography and measurement. It is important that no material is moved until these details have been recorded and the forensic dentist must follow instructions from the chief investigator and the pathologist. The dentist's main role at this point is not to carry out a complete forensic dental investigation but to determine whether there may be items such as dentures or crowns missing from the body for which a search must be made. If such items are found, their position in relation to the body should be recorded, they should be placed in labelled polythene bags, and should not be removed without the permission of the investigating officer.

1

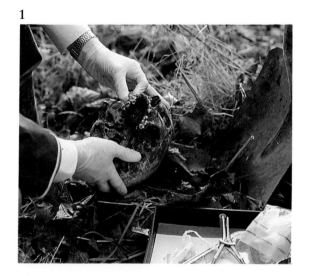

The dental identification kit

All necessary items should be kept available for instant use and consumables should be replaced as necessary.

2 Protective clothing. Most mortuaries will supply protective clothing for the dental examiner, but the kit should include a protective clean or sterile gown, rubber surgeon's gloves and heavy duty rubber gloves in varying sizes, a surgeon's cap and suitable masks. Because of the putrified nature of many bodies, masks incorporating activated charcoal or respirators should be available. The operator should wear protective spectacles or goggles. This is important where blood, serum or tissue fragments may be displaced into the atmosphere during removal of dental tissues, especially when an electric bone saw is used. The precautions usually taken in dental operating theatres or surgeries to prevent inhalation of aerosol or infected material will suffice.

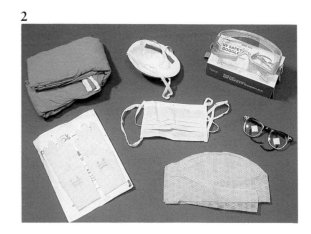

3 Dental instruments. Access to the oral cavity may present problems, and the kit should include lip retractors, tongue spatulae, rubber mouth props and a mouth gag of the forceps or screw type. Standard dental examination instruments will include mouth mirrors, tissue tweezers, both rat-toothed and smooth, dental probes of various designs, excavators and plastic instruments, swabs and cotton pledgets for cleaning the surfaces of the tissues. Surgical knives should include a selection of scalpel handles and disposable blades along with a heavy-duty post-mortem knife and one or more pairs of surgical scissors. A range of dental extraction forceps suitable for all types of tooth and a small selection of surgical elevators will frequently be useful. For cleansing and examination of the teeth toothbrushes and hand lenses may be needed.

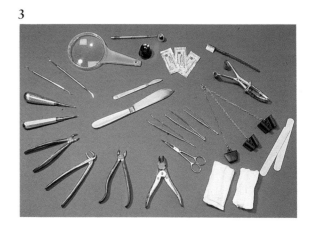

4 Impression materials. At each stage of the investigation the status of the oral cavity and teeth should be recorded, and this is most usually done following excision of the jaws. If this procedure cannot be carried out it may be necessary to take dental impressions. A selection of full and part mouth trays should be included. Alginate impressions will usually suffice, and packs of powder, measuring cylinders, rubber bowls and spatulae will be required. Warm water should be used to speed setting time in the absence of body heat. Where more accurate impressions are needed, silicone-type impression materials should be available. Soft dental wax may be used to record the normal occlusion, and suitable transport cases should be available to store impressions until they are cast. Disposable syringes are invaluable for the injection of impression materials into inaccessible areas.

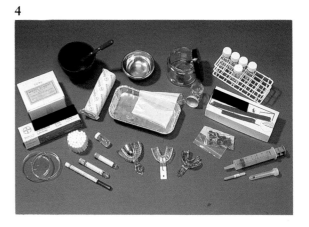

5

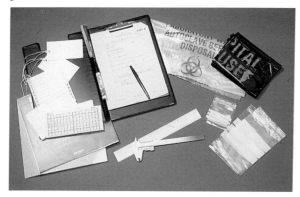

5 Recording the data. Data are best recorded by an assistant, or a dictaphone may be used, leaving the operator's hands free. The recording kit will include dental charts of various types, especially useful are those which portray all surfaces of all the teeth including the root surfaces and the position of gingival tissues and/or alveolar bone levels. Marker pens and pencils of various widths and colours and a clipboard and notepaper are essential. A selection of self-sealing plastic envelopes and self-adhesive or tie-on labels should be available, and it is useful to have pre-drawn outlines of the face and intra-oral structures so that the position, outline, size, extent and colour of any unusual features may be directly recorded. Pre-printed forms should be available to record the post-mortem findings so that ante-mortem findings, should they become available, may be easily compared. Along with the standard stationery and recording equipment, centimetre rules both rigid and flexible and a pair of adjustable calipers should be included. All of this equipment is best kept pre-packed in a suitable carrying case, one set kept at the place of work and one at the home of the investigator.

6

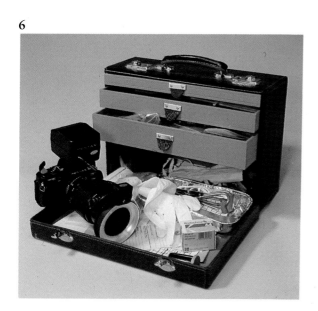

6 Photography. Many forensic dentists prefer their photography to be carried out by a professional hospital or police photographer, but this is not always possible and the kit should include a camera suitable for both extra-oral and intra-oral photography. A single lens reflex 35 mm camera with 100 mm focal length lens, exchangeable extension rings and ring-flash is usually adequate (but see **259**). It is important that a centimetre scale is included within the frame of the photograph but not obscuring any of the relevant detail. On flat surfaces the film plane of the camera is aligned as near parallel as possible to the subject, thus avoiding distortion, and two scales at right angles to each other should be inserted. On curved surfaces a rigid scale should be included in the frame. Plan views should be included in order that the relationships of particular items of interest to the surrounding structures may be appreciated. In addition to photography, tracings and labelled sketches of important features can be made on transparent overlays.

Examination of the body

In most cases the body will have been moved to the mortuary and a general post-mortem will have been carried out. The conditions of examination are usually therefore good with adequate lighting and the availability of general mortuary equipment. If a bite mark is present this should be studied before the general autopsy is carried out.

7 **Identification of the dead.** The dead are usually identified by facial recognition by a relative or acquaintance, and this may be possible even when only a part of the facial features is intact. We are all familiar with the recognition of well known personalities by contestants in television quiz shows and it is remarkable how accurate is our memory for unique facial features. Identification may be possible when only the eyes or the nose or part of the mouth is visible, but in such circumstances it may not be appropriate to subject the next-of-kin to unnecessary unpleasantness.

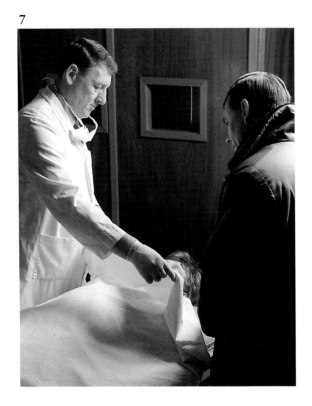
7

8 **General examination.** Two dentists should work together if possible, so that one can check the findings of the other. If death has recently occurred, or if the body has been preserved, then extra-oral examination is usually straightforward, but it may be necessary to turn the body so that all areas of the skin may be examined. There may be dental evidence, for example bite marks, which is more easily recognized by the forensic dentist. In the case of a putrescent or burnt corpse examination may be difficult but should be exhaustive even though the conditions may make this unpleasant.

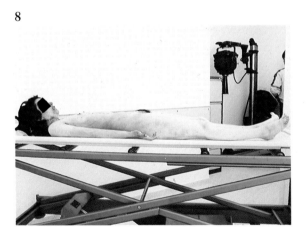
8

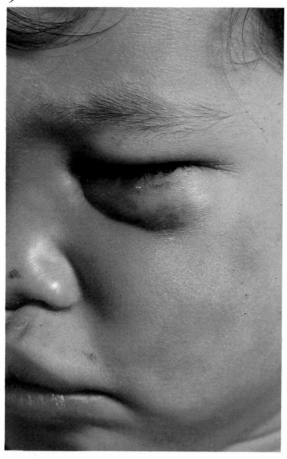

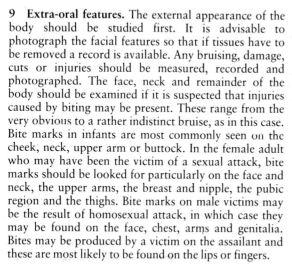

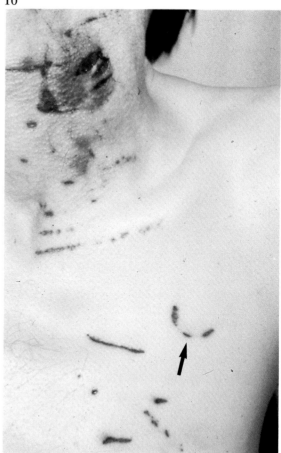

9   Extra-oral features. The external appearance of the body should be studied first. It is advisable to photograph the facial features so that if tissues have to be removed a record is available. Any bruising, damage, cuts or injuries should be measured, recorded and photographed. The face, neck and remainder of the body should be examined if it is suspected that injuries caused by biting may be present. These range from the very obvious to a rather indistinct bruise, as in this case. Bite marks in infants are most commonly seen on the cheek, neck, upper arm or buttock. In the female adult who may have been the victim of a sexual attack, bite marks should be looked for particularly on the face and neck, the upper arms, the breast and nipple, the pubic region and the thighs. Bite marks on male victims may be the result of homosexual attack, in which case they may be found on the face, chest, arms and genitalia. Bites may be produced by a victim on the assailant and these are most likely to be found on the lips or fingers.

10   Marks on the skin. Not all marks on the skin are caused by human bites. This man had been murdered by multiple knife wounds, and the injuries on the upper chest, especially the arcade-shaped mark (arrow), might be mistaken for a mark caused by human teeth. The dimensions of the arcade, the shape and the alignment of the marks precludes a bite from a human dentition, and the injury was probably caused by multiple stab wounds which coincidentally follow an arcade shape. Saliva swabs should be routinely taken if a bite is suspected, but marks which do not fit the patterns described in Chapter 14 are unlikely to be human bite marks. Such marks may be difficult to interpret and are best left to the forensic pathologist who will be experienced in non-bite mark injuries.

Intra-oral examination

When the examination of the whole body and especially the facial features has been completed the teeth, restorations, soft tissues, prostheses and jaws should be investigated.

11   The status of the teeth. The periodontal condition, including the level of the epithelial attachment, should be described because it will give some indication of the oral hygiene habits of the individual, and may also be useful in ageing techniques. Every surface of every tooth should be examined after cleansing, as the presence of composite restorations in particular may be missed under the often difficult conditions of examination. The manner in which the teeth occlude should be noted, along with any faceting caused by functional activity of the teeth. The distribution, colour and type of stains on the teeth should be noted as these may suggest the use of tobacco, beverages or medicaments. Mobility or fracture of any of the teeth or jaws may indicate that an assault has occurred.

12   The condition of the mouth. Debris, blood or soil may make recognition difficult and the teeth should be cleaned using a toothbrush and soapy water. Disclosing solutions may indicate the presence and boundaries of composite fillings in the anterior teeth. Photographs should be taken at each stage of the operation if there is a possibility of removal of evidence as the investigation proceeds. The cervical margins of the teeth should be inspected to indicate the presence of porcelain or acrylic crowns. If the oral tissues have been subjected to fire the materials from which crowns are constructed may react quite differently to the enamel of the natural teeth, making their presence more obvious. Care should be taken during the investigation to avoid displacing loose restorations or restorations damaged by excessive heat. The mercury in amalgams may vaporize when subjected to heat leaving a restoration in a powdery condition.

13   Charting the findings. As these details are determined they should be recorded on a standard dental chart. This anatomical type is probably the most useful because not only are occlusal, labial and lingual surfaces portrayed but the conditions of the roots and surrounding bone can be recorded diagrammatically. The presence of a dentally trained assistant is invaluable because the charting can be carried out under hygienic conditions without the need for the operator to transfer his attention continuously from the oral cavity to the charting table. When the dentist is single-handed, most of the information may be recorded on a suitably placed dictaphone. The information should be transferred to a dental chart as soon as possible and in the presence of the body as there may be no further opportunity to check the accuracy of the recording. The FDI two-digit system is shown here (see **193**).

11

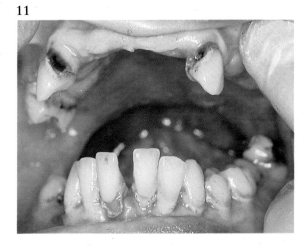

12

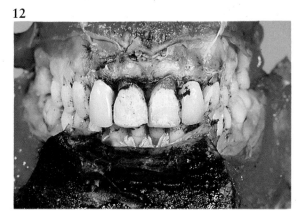

13

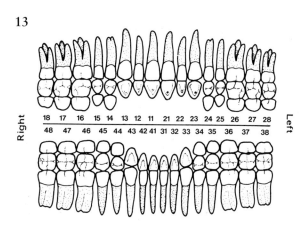

Right

18	17	16	15	14	13	12	11	21	22	23	24	25	26	27	28
48	47	46	45	44	43	42	41	31	32	33	34	35	36	37	38

Left

Skeletons and radiographs

Skeletonized remains provide the easiest access for dental examination. The skull and mandible are readily transportable and can be studied in the laboratory (**112** to **130**). The teeth and surrounding bone can be cleaned and it is unlikely that details of restorations will be incorrectly charted. It is easy to take satisfactory intra-oral and extra-oral radiographs and the specimen may be stored and later produced as evidence if necessary.

14

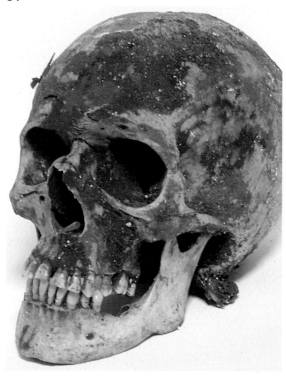

14 Surface debris on bones. Extraneous material on the surfaces of the bones should be collected. In this case an analysis of the soil covering the cranium revealed that the skull had previously been lying in a different environment, and had presumably been transported to the site at which it was found. There are recorded studies of barnacles being found attached to skull bones suggesting that at some time the body had been in a marine environment. Orifices in the skull such as the nasal cavity and the external auditory meatus may contain remnants of soil or sand and specimens of these should be retained for study by a soil analyst.

15

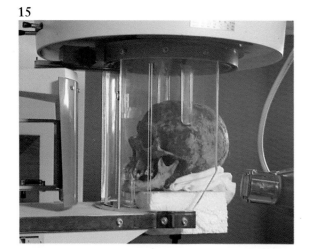

15 Radiographs of the jaws. These may take the form of intra-oral films covering the apices and crowns of all the teeth. If access is adequate, the jaws having been removed or the specimen skeletonized, occlusal films are useful to provide a scan view of the maxilla and the mandible. Because of the decomposed and unpleasant nature of many of the specimens requiring identification it is frequently inappropriate to transfer the body to the radiology department and the use of a portable machine in the mortuary may restrict the techniques available. Wherever the radiographs are taken, the equipment should be covered in plastic sheeting to avoid its contamination. Excised specimens should be fixed before radiography. Post-mortem radiographs may eventually be compared with ante-mortem radiographs and as many angulations as possible should be used so that like may be compared with like.

16 Identification from dental artefacts. Although fortunately not a common event, surgical artefacts may occasionally be left within the bony tissues. Examples are a fragment of amalgam incorporated into a healing socket, or in this case a surgical burr left at the site of removal of a wisdom tooth. It is incumbent on the surgeon to inform the patient of such an accident and to ensure that satisfactory radiographs are taken and a detailed description of the event placed in the medical notes. It may be that relatives of a person putatively identified have been told of a previous occurrence of this nature, but in any case dental surgeons should be contacted and their memories or records searched to provide comparative evidence leading to a positive identification. Useful information of this type will be missed unless routine radiographs are taken of every case.

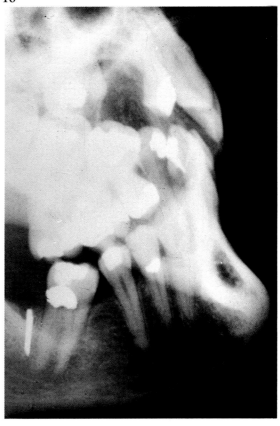

Chapter 3
Post-mortem procedures

The extra-oral examination of a body and the procedures to be followed when access to the oral cavity is straightforward have already been described in Chapter 2.

In most cases the forensic dentist is an invited specialist in the mortuary, and it is important that the usual courtesies are extended to the forensic pathologist who is in charge of the case. If the body has been stored or refrigerated it is most helpful to contact the mortuary in advance, giving an estimated time of arrival so that the body may be prepared for dental examination and the necessary assistance can be made available. If

possible, the dentist should attend with his own assistant who can help with retraction of tissues and with recording. In this situation, as in many others, two heads are often better than one. In most modern mortuaries the lighting is usually sufficient for an adequate examination to be made, but in some circumstances spotlights or additional angle-poise lights may be requested. The attendance at the mortuary should be arranged not only with the forensic pathologist but with the police in charge of the investigation and it is usual for an investigating officer to be present at the time.

Removal of post-mortem specimens

If it is necessary to remove specimens of either soft or hard tissue for further study, permission to do this must be obtained from the pathologist and from the coroner or

appropriate legal authority. This is especially important where the attendance of a defence expert may be necessary.

17

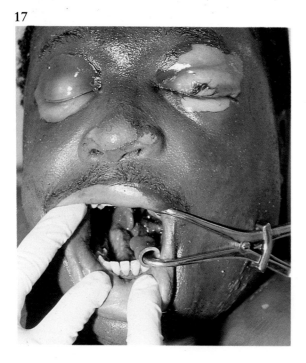

17 **Access to the mouth.** Immediately after death, before rigor is established and in some cases of moderate decomposition, it may be possible to open the jaws either manually or using the lever type of mouth gag. In both cases a rubber mouth prop should be inserted on the side opposite to that being examined to retain good access and visibility. This is possible in only a few cases, however and usually the teeth are held in tight occlusion. Forcible attempts to gain access to the oral cavity in these cases will almost certainly result in damage to some of the teeth or their restorations, and this approach should not be attempted. In any event, accurate charting may be difficult and it is usually better to remove the jaws.

18 Preparation for removal of the jaws. In many cases access to the oral cavity can be achieved only by removal of both upper and lower jaws. This has the added advantage that the hard tissues may be studied at leisure following suitable cleaning, radiographs can easily be taken, and specimens can be retained for presentation in court should this be necessary. Removal of the jaws will require saw cuts through the mandibular rami and the maxilla, and whether this is to be done using a hand or electric saw, infected material will inevitably be displaced from the body and the operator should wear a surgical mask and protective goggles or a visor so that no material is inhaled.

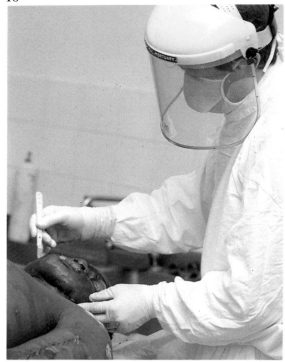

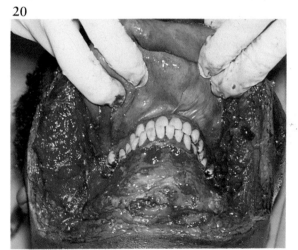

19 Initial incision. The preferred method of gaining access to the oral cavity, especially in cases where the body may be viewed, is a technique that involves minimal damage to the facial features. We would recommend that this technique be used in every case, as it is no more difficult technically than other methods of approach and the facial features can be retained with virtually no change. A horse-shoe incision is made below the lower border of the mandible and extending from the angle to the midline. Sharp dissection through the fatty and muscle tissues of the neck exposes the lower border of the mandible. The dissection continues outside the mandibular base so that the soft tissues can be stripped from the lateral and anterior surfaces of the mandible in an upward direction towards the vestibular attachment.

20 Exposure of the mandible. The attachment of the masseter muscles over the left and right mandibular rami must be incised at this stage, and the soft tissues of the chin can then be retracted upwards exposing the labial and anterior regions of the mandible until the vestibular attachment of the oral mucosa is reached. This can be incised, leaving the soft tissues of the attached gingivae intact. The soft tissues can be drawn up over the nasal region, exposing both upper and lower teeth, and the lateral and anterior surface of the mandible as far back as the retromolar region can be exposed, allowing access to the mandibular bone behind the last molar tooth.

21

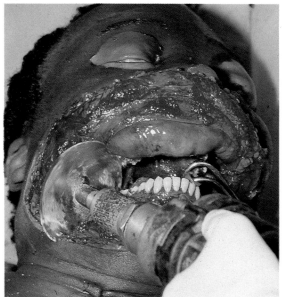

21 Sectioning the ramus. This dissection from the submandibular region will provide access to the labial and buccal surfaces of both the mandibular and maxillary teeth. It is completed by an incision through the labial vestibule in the maxilla, thus allowing the skin flap to be drawn up over the nasal region. The anterior nasal spine and the nasal apertures can be exposed in this way and the mandible may be readily removed by cutting through the ramus behind the lower third molar tooth. This saw cut is most safely done in a horizontal plane to the posterior margin of the mandible. In this case an oblique cut had to be made but this carries the risk of damage to the apices of a horizontal impacted wisdom tooth.

22

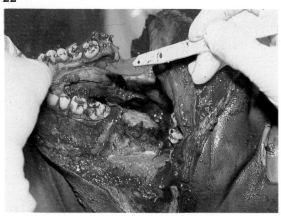

22 Excision of the mandible. The mandible can now be drawn downwards away from the maxilla and the soft tissues on the lingual side can be incised leaving the tongue and muscles of the floor of the mouth intact. This lingual incision can be extended below the lower border of the mandible on both sides, thus allowing it to be removed in one piece without damage to the teeth or supporting structures. This technique is much easier than attempting to dissect the muscles so that the condylar head can be disarticulated from the glenoid fossa, but this may be necessary if pathological changes are suspected in this part of the mandible.

23

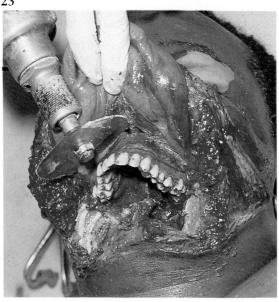

23 Sectioning the maxilla. Once the mandible has been removed a cut can be made using an electric saw above the level of the apices of all the teeth. The cut is made through the anterior nasal spine and the lateral wall of the maxillary antrum and, if possible, as far posteriorly as the pterygoid plates. It is important to retain the apices of the teeth because age estimations require a study of the apical part of each tooth, and the presence of root canal therapy may need to be compared with ante-mortem radiographs.

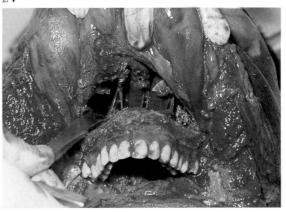

24 Removing the maxilla. Once the saw cut has been made through the bone on the lateral and anterior aspects of the maxilla the whole of the tooth-bearing area of this bone may be displaced downwards using a bone chisel with T-bar attachment. It is technically difficult to cut through all of the attachments of the tooth-bearing part of the maxilla, so a degree of force may be required to separate the maxillary region entirely from the pterygoid plates and the nasal septum. Once these have been fractured soft tissue attachments of the buccinator muscle, the pterygoid muscles and the muscles of the palate can be incised and the maxilla removed in one piece.

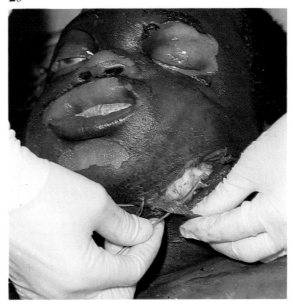

25 Replacement of soft tissues. Removal of most of the mandible and maxilla leaves a massive defect in the support of the soft tissues of the face. This can be dealt with satisfactorily by inserting gauze packing into the oral cavity in sufficient quantity to support the upper and lower labial regions, and arranging it to support the soft tissues of the chin. The soft tissues can be drawn down to the submandibular area and the skin sutured below the position of the lower border of the mandible, where it is unobtrusive in the unlikely event that the body has to be viewed.

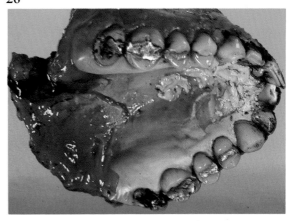

26 Cleaning the specimens. The excised maxilla and mandible can be studied in the mortuary and loose debris is easily removed by simple washing using a sponge and water. If the oral cavity is extensively covered with debris and burnt material it may be necessary to use a toothbrush and detergent solution. If more active agents such as hydrogen peroxide are to be used, the maxilla and mandible should first be photographed in colour, as bleaching of both hard and soft tissues may occur. Care should be taken at this stage to avoid dislodging fractured or loose portions of teeth or restorations, and if this should occur, their exact position should be recorded on a sketch map and the fragments should be retained in individual sealed plastic bags suitably labelled and numbered.

Following incineration or attempted cremation the surface of any gold restorations may have become amalgamated by free mercury which has evaporated from adjacent fillings, rendering their recognition difficult. The amalgam coating should be scraped away so that a correct diagnosis can be made.

Examination of the specimens

The presence or absence of teeth, restorations, malalignment or rotation of individual teeth and the status of edentulous spaces should be assessed.

Burn victims

These can be particularly difficult to examine because of damage to and swelling of soft tissues in the oral region. Access is usually difficult without jaw removal and incineration may make detailed observation impossible.

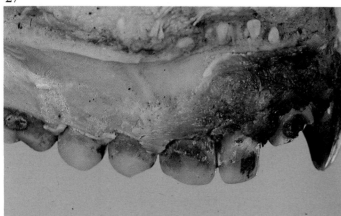

27 Anterior tooth restorations. This excised maxilla is from a burn victim. The upper right central incisor had broken off during the conflagration but the crown was discovered in the oral cavity. Following debridement and cleaning with a toothbrush and detergent the anterior teeth were inspected and probed for the presence or otherwise of anterior tooth-coloured restorations. Some authorities have suggested the use of phthalein dye, tinted benzalkonium chloride or aniline dyes to disclose the presence of silicate, plastic or quartz composite fillings, but they may also stain organic debris and plaque on the teeth. Tooth-coloured anterior fillings are often the most difficult features to establish, and visual examination alone may be insufficient for this purpose.

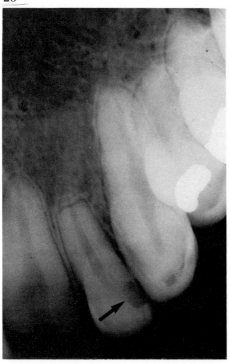

28 Confirmation by radiography. For the reasons outlined in caption **27**, it is wise routinely to radiograph anterior teeth, especially in the maxilla. This radiograph of the same burn victim as in **27** indicates the presence of a radiolucent filling material and the outline of a prepared cavity in the distal proximal surface of the upper left lateral incisor (arrow). If necessary, in doubtful cases the restorative material could be removed from the tooth of the victim and an analysis made of the material. The cheeks, tongue and to some extent the lips tend to protect the teeth if death occurred before a fire. If death occurs during a fire the lips are often drawn back exposing the anterior teeth.

29 Maceration of soft tissues. When the jaws have been removed from the body, colour photographs should be taken before further changes occur to the soft tissues or the colour. There are various ways of macerating the specimens. Some workers fix briefly in 10% formol saline and then dry the specimens. The dried soft tissue is then readily removed. Complete maceration is possible by simmering in 10% detergent solution followed by 5% hydrogen peroxide solution.

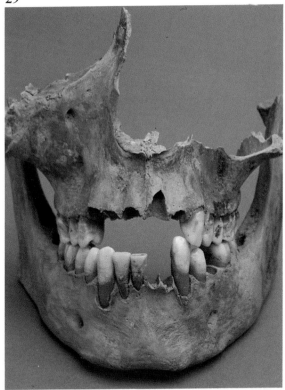

30 Checking the dental findings. Because of the problems encountered in dental examination in the mortuary it is advisable to recheck any findings on the macerated and prepared specimens. It is useful at this stage to have this second examination carried out by an independent investigator, thus checking the original findings and perhaps disclosing new information. Additional information from radiographs or specialized studies such as microscopy should be incorporated at this stage before the final report is written.

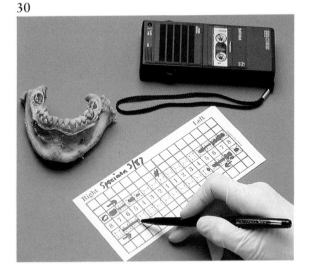

Impressions and excision of other specimens

There are occasions where parts of the body other than the oral cavity may need to be examined by the forensic dentist. The most common example is where human bite marks have been left on the skin. Following sketches, tracings and photography (see **232**) it is sometimes useful, especially if the skin has been penetrated, to take an accurate impression of the area. If histological study is required the skin may need to be excised.

31

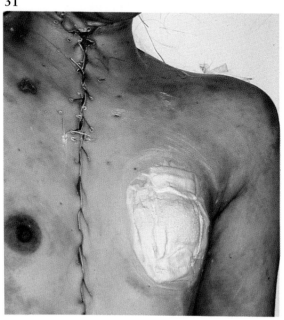

31 Preservation of the bite mark. In this case of rape and murder a human bite mark was left on the nipple and areola of the victim. Silicone rubber has been injected on to the area and the flexible impression has been backed with strips of plaster of Paris to provide rigidity. Histological study was necessary to prove that the tissue damage was compatible with that expected in a human bite (see **190**) and in these circumstances an excision including a wide area of normal tissue should be made. Distortion during fixation can be minimized by suturing the specimen over a preformed mould the shape of the original supporting tissues.

Chapter 4
Tooth status and arrangement

Because the teeth are the most indestructible part of the body, they are likely to remain following the loss of soft tissues by putrefaction or dissolution. Their number and individuality of shape and content may be the only way of determining identity when other features have long disappeared. Although the human adult dentition comprises 32 teeth, eight in each quadrant, one or more teeth may be absent because of failure to develop or because of subsequent loss before or after death. The teeth that are present may have unusual characteristics of size, shape or surface contour, and they may have been changed by environmental conditions which reflect the lifestyle of their owner. The arrangement of the teeth within the upper and lower arches may be regular or irregular so that people who have never attended a dental surgeon may still have sufficient idiosyncrasies in their teeth to enable them to be identified. The forensic dentist should be capable of recognizing individual teeth when present in the mouth or when only single teeth or fragments are available. In an Atlas of this nature it is not possible to include examples of all the abnormalities which may occur in the human dentition. The information should be sought in texts of oral pathology.

In practice, the status of the teeth is usually studied in cases of identification but may also become important if human bite marks appear to have been produced by an abnormal dentition.

Arrangement of teeth

The forensic dentist, in charting the teeth present in the mouth, needs to be aware of the nuances of shape which each tooth possesses. In most cases the teeth are arranged in a pattern which is the same in all human beings and consists of incisors at the anterior part of the mouth, a canine separating the incisors from the premolars and the molars, which are grinding teeth, being placed posteriorly in the arch.

32

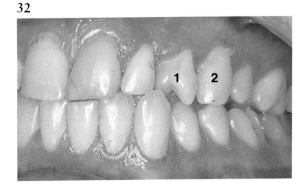

32 The position of the teeth. Teeth may be transposed so that their order in the arch is abnormal, and this event is so rare that this feature alone may result in positive identification. In this case, the first premolar (1) has been transposed with the upper canine (2). The incidence of minor or major variations in tooth position or angulation have been calculated statistically from studies of large populations.

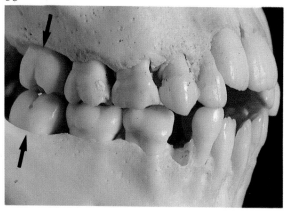

33

33 Deciduous and permanent teeth. During development of the dentition a stage is reached where both deciduous and permanent teeth are present in the mouth. This stage is known as the mixed dentition and occurs between the ages of six years and around twelve years. It is essential to be able to distinguish between the deciduous and permanent teeth, so a sound knowledge of tooth morphology is a prerequisite for the forensic dentist. In this specimen the first permanent molars (arrows) have erupted behind the deciduous molars, which are still in function, and the upper and lower permanent incisors are replacing their deciduous predecessors. This indicates an age of about six and a half to seven years.

Teeth not present in the arch

Having assessed the teeth which are present in the mouth, the next stage is to determine which are missing and the reason for their absence. In the younger person the most likely reason for absence of a tooth is that it has not yet clinically erupted. Other possibilities are that the tooth has been extracted or has not developed at all.

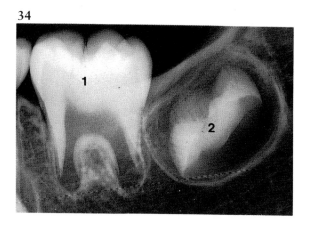

34

34 Unerupted teeth. In this radiograph the first permanent molar (1) is present but the second molar (2) is incomplete and unerupted. A study of the degree of development of the roots of these teeth enables an estimate of age to be made. In this example the roots of the first molar have completed about two-thirds of their development, and the crown of the second molar is about two-thirds complete, indicating an age of about six years.

The stage of development of the dentition at a particular age will vary somewhat from individual to individual. Estimates are therefore of biological age rather than chronological age. Development of teeth is often more advanced in girls than in boys of the same age.

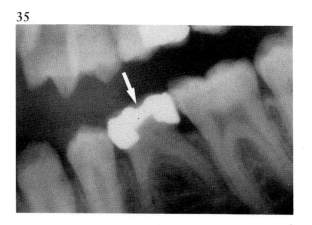

35

35 Developmentally missing teeth. Teeth may be missing because they have never developed. In this example the lower second premolar is absent and its predecessor, the second deciduous molar (arrow) has been retained. It was important in this case that the forensic dentist recognized the heavily filled second deciduous molar for what it was, and radiographs will help towards a correct diagnosis. The most commonly absent tooth, apart from the third molar, is said to be the mandibular second premolar, followed by the maxillary second premolar and the maxillary second incisor.

36 Teeth lost before and after death. The absence of a tooth in an unidentified body when compared with the ante-mortem dental records does not rule out an identification. It is, however, necessary to be able to determine whether the tooth was lost before or after death. If the margins of the empty tooth socket are sharp and unresorbed, as in this case, the tooth was probably lost after death. Resorption and remodelling of the socket margins would indicate that the tooth had been lost before death. Further details of the method are described in Chapter 6.

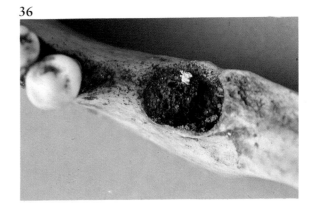

Additional or malshaped teeth

Teeth of unusual shape, size or number are sufficiently rare to be useful in identification procedures, as they will have been noted in ante-mortem records.

37 Supernumerary teeth. In this example there is an erupting supernumerary incisor (arrow) present in the palate. About two per cent of people have supernumerary teeth of one type or another and there is evidence that they occur most frequently in the microdont black races. The commonest site of an additional tooth is in the maxillary incisor region and the tooth may be conical or tuberculate in shape. One or more of these teeth in the midline are often referred to as a mesiodens. The bilateral occurrence of additional molar teeth is not uncommon in coloured races.

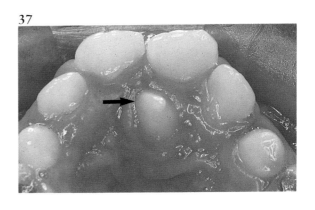

38 Additional cusps. Any unusual form of the teeth may be a useful identification feature. The central incisors are developmentally derived from three mineralization centres, so that the incisal edge (before it becomes worn) shows three tubercles or mamelons. It is sometimes difficult to draw the line between a variation within normal limits and a definite abnormality, but in this specimen there is an additional cusp on the labial surface of the upper left central incisor which is a very unusual feature. Frequently, when additional cusps are present there may be a hereditary factor, so investigations of the family may be worthwhile.

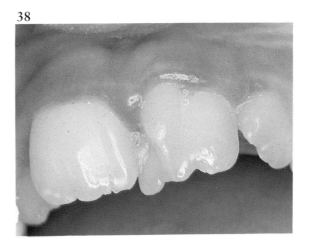

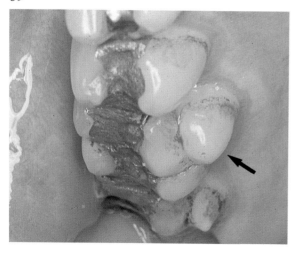

39 The cusp of Carabelli. Not all additional cusps can be regarded as abnormalities and on most upper first molars there is a groove or ledge on the palatal side of the mesiopalatal cusp (arrow). In about 50 per cent of Europeans this may be exaggerated into an additional cusp known as the cusp of Carabelli. The presence of this cusp in an unknown body may provide some clue as to the racial origin of the individual. Other racially related oral characteristics include arch width, midline diastema, enamel pearls, shape and size of incisors, cuspal patterns in molars, the shape of the mandible and maxilla and the presence of bony excrescences or tori in both mandible and maxilla. Comprehensive reviews of racial and hereditary characteristics are available in the literature.

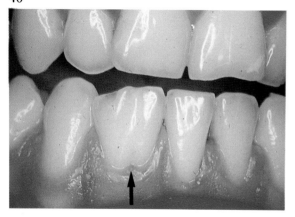

40 Fused or geminated teeth. A sufficiently unusual feature to be useful in identification procedures is the presence of fused teeth. This process is known as gemination and it may be caused during development. In this example the lower right central and lateral incisors have fused (arrow). Another cause of gemination or twinning of teeth is the deposition of large amounts of cementum around the roots of two adjacent teeth. This is not true gemination and is usually referred to as false gemination. The commonest site for this occurrence is pathological fusion between the upper second and third molars.

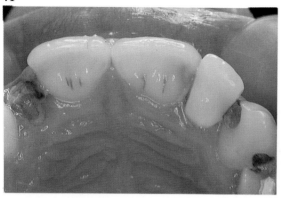

41 Macrodontia. The size of the teeth is usually roughly related to the size of the cranium, and whilst there is considerable racial variation the relationship usually falls within quite narrow limits. Occasionally extremely large or small teeth are seen, termed macro- or microdontia. In this example the upper central incisors are much wider than would be expected from the size of the dental arch. The teeth most frequently affected are the maxillary first incisor and canine, and sometimes the mandibular second premolar and third molar. The incidence is rare enough to be useful in identification procedures.

Hereditary conditions and malocclusions

The structure of the teeth and their position in the mouth may be modified by hereditary conditions that result in defective hard tissue formation or bone relationships. Some malocclusions may also be dependent upon local factors.

42 Amelogenesis and dentinogenesis. Certain inherited disorders may present as defects in the teeth. For example, the enamel may be affected in amelogenesis imperfecta, and the dentine is imperfectly formed in dentinogenesis imperfecta. There are also variants of amelogenesis imperfecta, and diagnosis of a specific type may make identification even more certain. Dentinogenesis imperfecta may also be of differing expression, one type being associated with osteogenesis imperfecta, whilst others are not, perhaps being of racial significance. In this example of dentinogenesis imperfecta brittle bone disease was also present. The crowns of the teeth are bulbous and the enamel has chipped away from the defective dentine. These conditions have a familial background and families with these genetic abnormalities are usually well documented. Recognition of such conditions may be of help both in identification and in paternity cases.

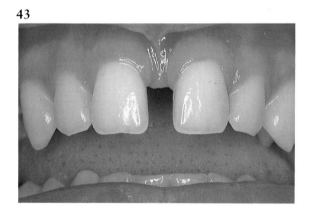

43 Diastema. Midline diastema is said to be more common in Australian Aborigines, South African Ostraloid and Boskopoid peoples and is rare in Bantu and Bushmen. The condition is sufficiently striking to be useful as an identification pointer because relatives and acquaintances would be aware of even minor abnormalities at the front of the mouth, whereas gross abnormalities in the posterior region may pass unnoticed. Bite marks produced by dentitions possessing a diastema may demonstrate this striking feature.

44 Malocclusions. Because the incidence of malplaced teeth may be high in a given community, only gross malocclusions may be useful in identification procedures, although in a mass disaster, where names and dental records of many of the victims may be available, it may be useful to include descriptions of the occlusion of the teeth as each body is examined. Malocclusions have been classified according to whether the jaws have a normal relationship and the teeth are misplaced, or whether the relationship of maxilla to mandible is disturbed. Only striking malocclusions such as this may be useful in identification procedures.

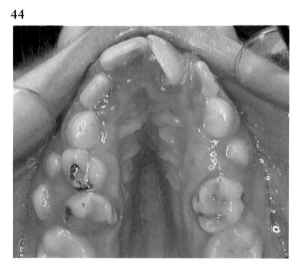

Unusual wear and trauma

Some dentitions have been extensively modified by contact with opposing teeth, foreign bodies or by impact. The patterns so produced may be sufficiently unusual to help in identification procedures.

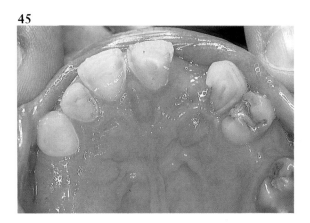

45

45   Tooth attrition. Severe attrition of the teeth may be caused by unusual occlusions, abnormal functional loads or by continuous grinding of the teeth in conditions such as bruxism. Attrition patterns will also indicate the presence or absence of opposing teeth in bodies where the mandible has been lost as a result of putrefaction. The state of the dentition during life may therefore to some extent be determined even when only one jaw is available. Men usually exhibit more attrition than women at a given age and so the phenomenon may aid in sex determination. The degree of wear is dependent upon the type of diet, and may be severe as a result of habits such as tobacco chewing and in occupations in which workers are exposed to atmospheres containing abrasive dust.

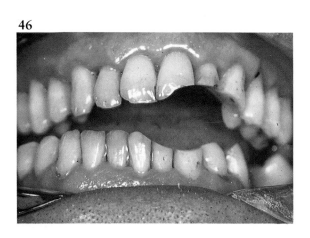

46

46   Occupational habits. Certain habits and occupations may leave a permanent mark on the dentition enabling the forensic dentist to comment upon these aspects of a person's life. This severe and characteristic pattern of wear was seen in a bagpipe player. Notching of the upper central or lateral incisors has been frequently described in hairdressers who may habitually hold hairclips in the mouth before transferring them to their client's hair (see **149**). Typical abrasion may also occur in such trades as carpentry or shoe repairing where the craftsman may hold a number of nails between the teeth before transferring them to the workpiece. Habitual pipe smokers may produce characteristic patterns of wear.

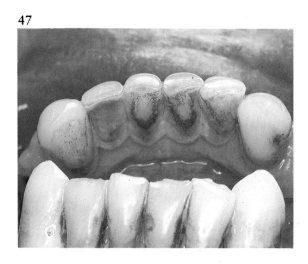

47

47   Erosion of teeth. More generalized changes to the teeth can sometimes result from nutritional habits such as excessive ingestion of beverages with a low pH, and this particular case of generalized erosion was attributed to a high daily intake of beer. Erosion is removal of tooth tissue by means of chemical activity other than that caused by micro-organisms in the mouth. The defects are usually smooth, scooped-out depressions frequently on the labial and buccal cervical margins of the teeth. Most often several teeth are involved and the cause may not be apparent. Chronic vomiting, the use of acidic drinks or citrus fruits may be implicated. It has been reported that young women with anorexia nervosa may suffer from this condition because of regurgitation of gastric contents and the intake of unsatisfactory diets. The lip aspect of the lower teeth shown here lies below a mirror view of their tongue aspect.

48 Tooth fracture. A common cause of change in the position or shape of a tooth is trauma. This may result in displacement and non-vitality of teeth or in fracture, displaced or otherwise, of bones of the face. Evidence of healing may be visible in the teeth and facial skeleton for a considerable time after the event and may be useful in identification procedures. Abnormality of the front teeth caused by untreated trauma may be important in the analysis of a bite mark inflicted during an attack on a victim (see **237**).

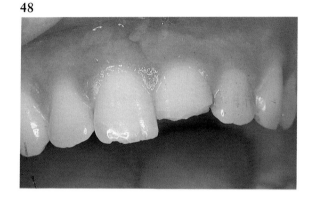

48

Tooth defects and pigmentation

There are said to be more than 30 general disorders of health which may manifest themselves in the oral cavity, and some workers have recorded more than 50 systemic diseases producing signs in good radiographs taken of the teeth and jaws. As far as the teeth are concerned, a number of generalized conditions, especially those present at the time of their development, may produce permanent defects or marks in the enamel or dentine.

49 Hypoplastic teeth. Childhood conditions such as whooping cough, mumps or measles may produce hypoplasia at the relevant time in the stage of development of the enamel and such defects have figured as vital evidence in at least one murder trial in the United Kingdom. Localized infections may involve only one developing tooth, but generalized systemic conditions will affect the part of each tooth developing at the time of the disturbance. Defects such as these seen in the upper incisor teeth will therefore not only indicate childhood illness but may enable the forensic dentist to determine exactly at what age the disturbance occurred. This may be useful if previous medical records can be traced.

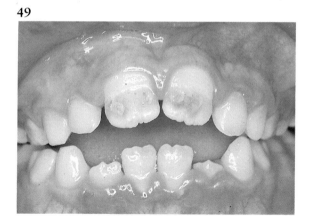

49

50 Ante-mortem pink teeth. Changes in the colour of the teeth may be indicative of activity within the tooth, or in some cases external pigmentation. Texts of oral medicine are a more appropriate place to discuss the differential diagnosis. This example is of internal resorption of the structure of the tooth resulting in the vascular pulp becoming visible through the labial surface of the upper right incisor. The condition provides one example of a 'pink' tooth. Pink teeth are also a well known post-mortem finding of forensic importance (see **183** and **184**).

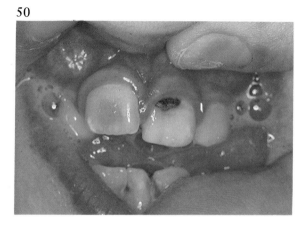

50

Chapter 5
Tooth restorations

Identification by dental means is dependent upon the individuality of different people's mouths. While the number of teeth present and features of their size, shape and arrangement may be sufficiently distinctive to allow identification, it is more often the detailed consideration of dental treatment evident in a mouth which leads to identification.

The most frequently useful evidence of dental treatment is restorative work. In this chapter the range of dental restorative procedures in current use is illustrated. Consideration is then given to some of the problems that can be encountered in identifying these in situations such as badly burned bodies or where other damage has occurred to restorations.

Tooth restoration is required because of loss of tooth substance by decay (dental caries), fracture of a tooth, or the abnormal wearing away of teeth for a variety of reasons. Of these, restorations replacing areas damaged by dental caries are the most frequent, and can involve single or multiple surfaces of individual teeth. The full description of a restoration includes the material used and the surfaces restored.

Restorative dental techniques

51

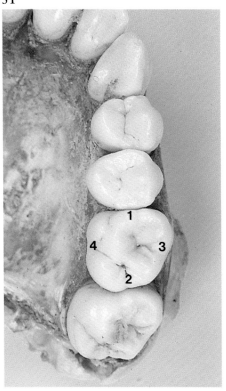

51 Nomenclature of surfaces of posterior teeth. Posterior teeth can be considered as having five surfaces. Any single surface or combination may have been subjected to restorative work. The biting surface is known as the occlusal surface. The other surfaces are designated mesial (1) distal (2) buccal (3), which is towards the cheek, and palatal (4) in the upper jaw (lingual in the lower jaw).

52 Nomenclature of fillings. Restorations are designated by the surface involved and the material used. Commonly, posterior teeth are restored by silver amalgam. The third molar (1), and the second molar (2) have occlusal amalgams. The first molar (3) has a mesio-occluso-palatal (MOP) amalgam and the second premolar (4) has a disto-occlusal (DO) amalgam.

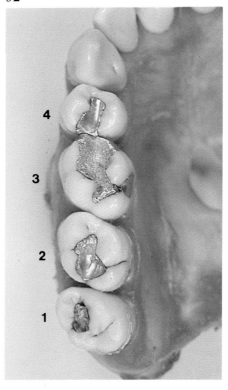

53 Further aspects of fillings. In this case the second molar tooth (arrow) shows an amalgam near the neck of the tooth on the buccal aspect. There is evidence of corrosion of this amalgam filling, indicating that it is likely to have been in place for some years. The amalgam filling in the adjacent first molar also involves the buccal aspect of the tooth but is in the form of an extension of the filling that also involves other tooth surfaces. This filling shows evidence of two episodes of treatment, in that the part nearer the gum has been restored at a different time, probably later, than the other part of the filling.

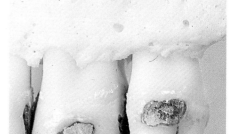

54 Temporary filling. For a variety of reasons it may not be possible or appropriate to place a permanent filling in a cavity at a particular time. In these circumstances the dentist may choose to fill a prepared cavity with a temporary dressing or filling. A variety of materials is used for this purpose. These are much less durable than permanent fillings, and if present will usually indicate a recent visit to the dentist, with treatment in progress. In the case illustrated, an MOD cavity has been temporarily filled with a dental cement.

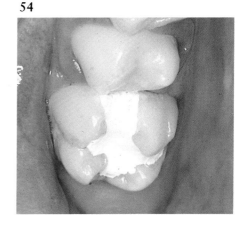

55

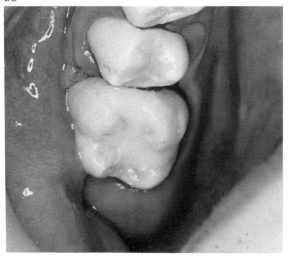

55 Tooth-coloured restorations. There is an increasing trend towards the use of tooth-coloured composite filling materials for posterior teeth in preference to amalgam. The illustration shows the same tooth as in **54** after the temporary filling has been replaced with a composite. Careful examination may be required to detect such fillings.

56

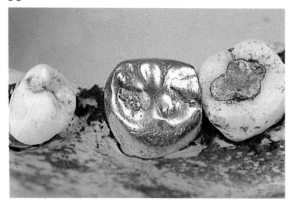

56 Gold crown. Extensively decayed teeth may be restored with a crown or cap. In this case a cast gold crown restores one molar tooth. The other molar tooth has an occlusal amalgam filling. The presence of more complex restorations such as crowns improves the chances of successful identification by dental means.

57

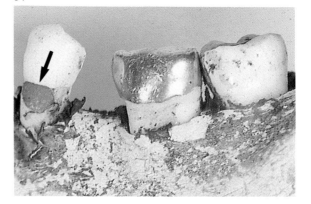

57 Gold crown and cervical amalgam. This view is of the cheek aspect of the teeth shown in **56**. It confirms that the gold restoration is a shell crown covering the whole crown of the tooth. In addition there is an amalgam filling in the cervical part of the premolar tooth (arrow). This is a type of filling found particularly in older people, where gum recession is followed by decay at the neck of the tooth.

58

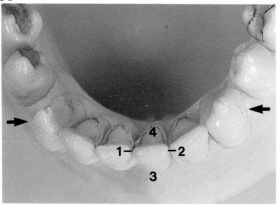

58 Nomenclature of anterior tooth surfaces. Anterior teeth can be considered as having four surfaces and a biting edge (the incisal edge). The four surfaces are the mesial surface (1) nearer the midline, the distal surface (2) further from the midline, the labial surface (3) opposed to the lips, and the lingual surface (4) adjacent to the tongue. In the upper jaw this is the palatal surface. Canine or eye teeth (arrows) show a variably pointed cusp rather than an incisal edge.

59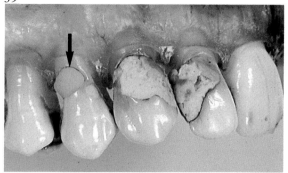

60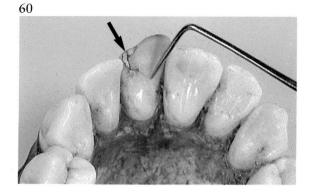

59 Anterior tooth-coloured fillings. Commonly, white filling materials are used at the front of the mouth. The cervical filling in the first premolar (arrow) is a reasonable match for the tooth colour. The restorations in the other two teeth are poor. Good composite fillings can be difficult to detect, especially if dental charting is undertaken in relatively poor lighting in the mortuary.

60 Recognition of tooth-coloured fillings. Some authorities recommend the use of various dyes to ensure that tooth-coloured fillings are detected. The black dye in this case does emphasize part of the margin of this filling (arrow). However, it is quicker and easier to detect fillings and determine their extent by the use of a sharp dental probe, because the texture differs from that of tooth enamel.

61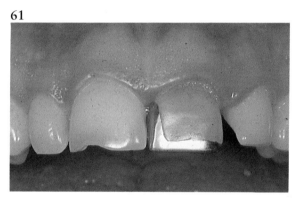

62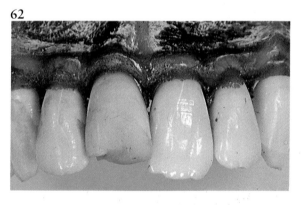

61 Anterior gold inlay. The upper left incisor has been restored with a gold inlay. This is used when the biting edge of the tooth has been damaged by fracture or decay. In this case the restored tooth is slightly darker than the adjacent teeth and also appears to have lost some of the natural translucency. This suggests that the nerve of the tooth may be dead. In such cases evidence of root treatment should be sought.

62 Acid etch restoration of incisal edge. Modern white filling materials can be used to attempt to restore the incisal edge. Here, an acid etch technique, followed by the use of a composite filling material, has been used in an unsuccessful attempt to restore a fractured incisal edge. This proved important in the identification of this boy whose death was accidental.

63

63 Anterior tooth crowns. The upper right central incisor (1) has been restored with a crown consisting of a non-precious metal backing and porcelain. The upper left central incisor (2) has been restored with a porcelain shell crown. A defect, or an area of recurrent decay at the neck of this tooth has been restored with amalgam.

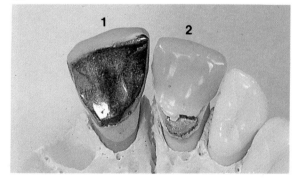

64

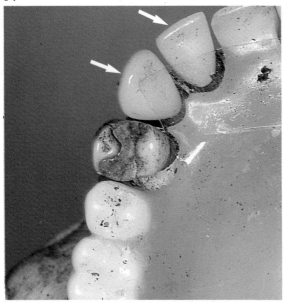

64 Porcelain crowns. The porcelain crowns (arrows) and acrylic maxillary denture were found in the skeletonized remains of a male body found in a wooded area. An important aspect of the investigation was to determine when the man had died. Analysis of the crowns revealed that the type of porcelain had been in use only for a relatively short period, and the crowns had been placed in the mouth not long before death. The estimated time of death was supported by the finding of both pre-decimal and decimal coins in a fragment of a pocket, suggesting that death had occurred around 1971.

65

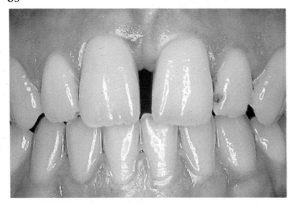

65 Marked alteration of tooth shape or appearance. With the advent of techniques of modifying the shapes and appearance of teeth by composite fillings or by bonded porcelain facings, dramatic changes in appearance can be achieved with much less restorative work than is required for crowns. This patient had an unsightly gap between the upper central incisors—a central diastema. Several techniques can be used to improve this.

66

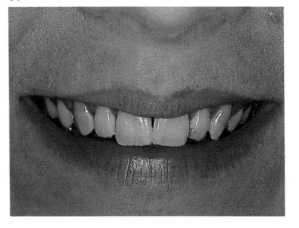

66 Correction of central diastema. This is the same patient as shown in **65**. The shape of the two upper central incisors has been altered by the addition of small porcelain bonded facings covering only parts of the teeth. These can be difficult to detect even on careful clinical examination. In cases where 'toothy snapshots' are being used to supplement ante-mortem dental records, as described in **207**, the possibility of such dramatic alterations in tooth shape by restorative procedures must be borne in mind.

Advanced restorative dentistry

With improvements in oral hygiene and dental care in developed countries many more adults retain their teeth into old age. Accompanying this change there has been a substantial increase in the use of more elaborate and complex techniques for tooth restoration and the replacement of missing teeth.

67

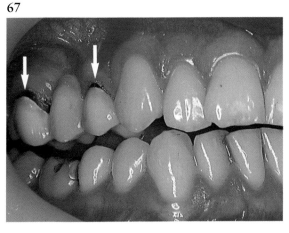

68

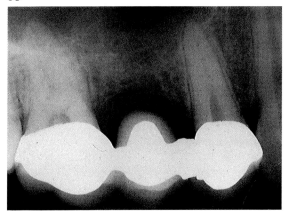

67 Tooth replaced by bridge. This patient had a well cared for mouth, but extraction of a tooth had left her with an unsightly gap. The missing tooth has been replaced by a pontic with the visible areas consisting of porcelain closely matching the shade of the other teeth. In order to support the pontic, crowns made of gold and porcelain (arrows) have been placed upon the adjacent teeth.

68 Radiograph of bridge. The radiograph of the bridge shown in **67** confirms that crowns have been placed on vital teeth on either side of the gap caused by the missing tooth. The metal core of the porcelain-faced pontic is also clearly evident.

Endodontic treatment

If the tooth pulp is damaged by extension of dental decay or by exposure when a tooth is fractured, it may be necessary to remove the pulp and insert a root canal filling in order to retain the tooth. The pulp of the tooth is exposed sufficiently to allow the soft tissues to be removed by instrumentation of the root canal. The root canal is enlarged and if necessary sterilized. A root filling is then placed and the crown of the tooth is restored using one of the techniques already described. The presence of root canal fillings is demonstrated by radiographs of the teeth.

69

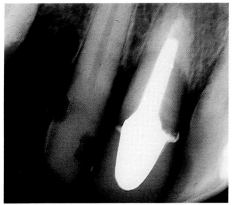

69 Root-treated anterior tooth. The crown of the upper right central incisor had been extensively destroyed by decay. The pulp of the tooth has been removed and the root canal enlarged to allow a root filling to be inserted. The root canal also supports a cast metal post, the purpose of which is to reform part of the crown of the tooth. The final restoration would be an artificial crown made of acrylic or porcelain such as that shown in **63**.

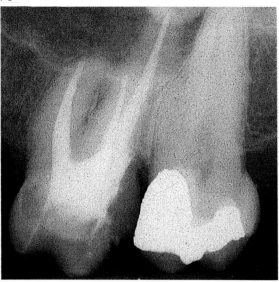

70 Root-treated posterior tooth. Molar teeth have multiple root canals and are less often root treated. This radiograph shows the radiopaque root fillings in the root canals. When the crown of the tooth has been restored it is not possible to detect the presence of root fillings without the use of radiographs.

Recognition of restorative dental work

If the fillings are missing from teeth in a body it is important to be able to recognize that a cavity has been caused by dental treatment. In instances where the teeth have been damaged at death or following death this can be difficult to ascertain.

71

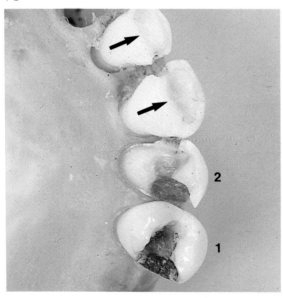

72

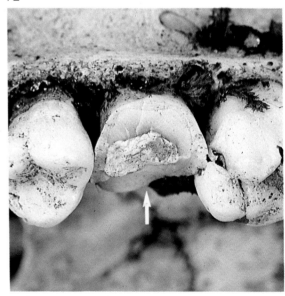

71 Recognition of cavities. It is important to be able to distinguish areas of tooth loss caused by cavity preparation from loss resulting from other causes. The premolar tooth (1) and the canine tooth (2) show cavities on the distal aspects from which fillings are missing. The loss of tooth substance in other teeth (arrows) was caused by attrition, where the lower teeth had been wearing against these upper teeth.

72 Evidence of restoration in damaged teeth. This body had been on open moorland for a considerable time after death. Many of the teeth had cracked and split, probably as a result of freezing. The crown of the second molar tooth (arrow) has broken off, but it is still possible to identify that there had been an occlusal filling in the tooth. The remaining restorative material is the lining which was placed beneath an amalgam filling.

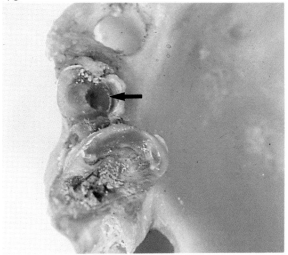

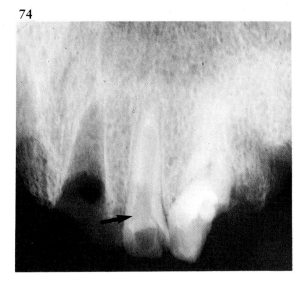

73 Recognition of restorative work. In this body, which was recovered from the sea, many of the teeth were missing, having fallen out after death. Some of the remaining teeth appeared badly broken down. However, closer examination revealed that the root canals were larger than normal (arrow) and were round rather than oval in shape. This suggested that the teeth might have been root treated.

74 Evidence of root canal instrumentation. Radiographs of the teeth in the case shown in 73 confirmed that the root canals had been enlarged by instrumentation. The shape of the root canal in the first premolar (arrow) indicates that it has been used to support a metal post, such as that shown in **69**. In fact the teeth, far from being broken down by neglect, had been root treated and restored by crowns—evidence of substantial dental treatment.

Recognition of cremated restorations

Fragments of teeth may remain in the debris associated with a prolonged fire and may be the only recognizable portion of a body.

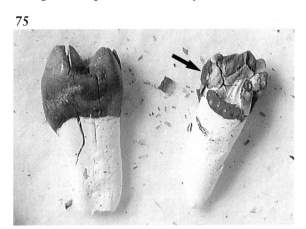

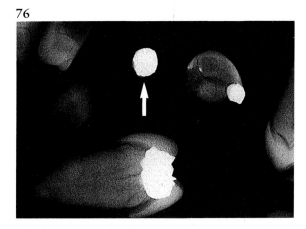

75 Teeth incinerated at 600°C. The roots of the teeth have undergone marked colour changes and these may give a broad indication of the temperature reached during the fire. In this case they have a chalky white appearance and may be extremely friable, so care is needed to retrieve and examine them. A piece of amalgam (arrow) is still visible in the fragmented tooth crown on the right.

76 Radiographs of fragments. In cases where tooth fragments cannot easily be distinguished amongst other debris, a radiograph will often be useful. Enamel and dentine may be recognizable, as are the fragments of amalgam (arrow).

Chapter 6
The bones of the skull (including the jaws)

Apart from victims of fire or drowning, most bodies requiring identification will have become unrecognizable because extensive putrefaction has occurred, eventually resulting in skeletonization of the remains. In the nature of things, bodies requiring the attention of the dental surgeon are frequently discovered in isolated areas, and a considerable time has usually elapsed since death. The body will have been exposed to the elements, to putrefaction, and to the attack of insects and wildlife. Following bacterial attack and the attention of scavengers, the soft tissues are lost and eventually the bones themselves may become disarticulated, damaged and dispersed. The environment causes changes in bones, and the rate at which these changes occur is extremely variable depending upon the site at which the body is found.

The forensic dentist is trained and experienced in the examination and interpretation of the teeth, and much of this Atlas is inevitably concentrated on this particular area. At first sight it may be thought that the anatomist or physical anthropologist is best equipped to deal with skeletal remains, but dental science is concerned not only with the development and structure of the teeth but also with the supporting structures, notably the jaws. Collaborative studies between the anthropologist, anatomist, forensic pathologist and dentist have been fruitful, particularly in studies of large populations from ancient times, as well as in investigations with forensic implications. Numerous cases have arisen where unusual features of the bones, such as sites of healed fractures or other bone diseases, have confirmed the medical history of a particular person. The post-cranial parts of a skeleton may be important in these respects and may initially provide some information on the forensic significance of the remains and the amount of time likely to have elapsed since death.

The presence of long bone cartilages or remnants of ligaments would indicate that death occurred fairly recently, whereas erosion, pitting, chalkiness and staining of the bones may indicate that much of the protein content has been lost, and that the bones are not of recent origin. Post-cranial parts of the skeleton, particularly the pelvis, sacrum or long bones may give some indication of the sex of the person, and the extent of ossification of the epiphyses provides a standard method for ageing the younger skeleton at the time of death. Racial characteristics may sometimes be determined from the pelvis and femur, and formulae can be used to calculate stature from the long bones, particularly the femur and tibia and, less accurately, the fibula and bones of the arm. The forensic dentist rarely has sufficient experience in post-cranial skeletal structures to claim expertise in this field.

We have sought to restrict this Atlas as far as possible to matters which unarguably fall within the province of the forensic dentist, and for this reason only the information to be gained from a study of the bones of the skull is included. Aspects of age determination from the skull bones are discussed. However, the determination of age at death from a study of the embryology, eruption status and later changes in the dentition are covered in Chapter 8.

Determination of age from the skeleton

Estimates of age from biological material cannot strictly be equated with chronological age because of the variation in development that occurs between different individuals. Reasonable estimates, however, can be made from a study of the bones of the skull. The forensic dentist is rarely called upon to examine fetal material, though it has been shown that a reasonably accurate estimate of age can be made from measurements of individual fetal skull bones. More frequenly, cases will be in the neonatal or circumnatal period.

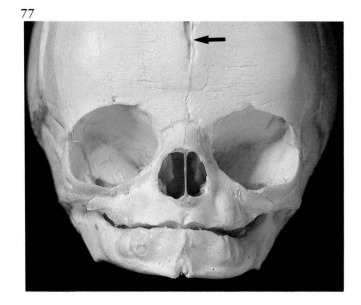

77 Neonatal skull. In this neonatal skull the lack of eruption of the dentition places the age at less than six months after birth. The height of the face is small compared with an older child, whereas the relative size of the orbits is large. In most infants the midline symphysis of the mandible is fused by about one year after birth, and the lack of fusion in this specimen indicates a much lower age. The metopic suture (arrow) between the two halves of the frontal bone fuses at about one year, but there are racial variations.

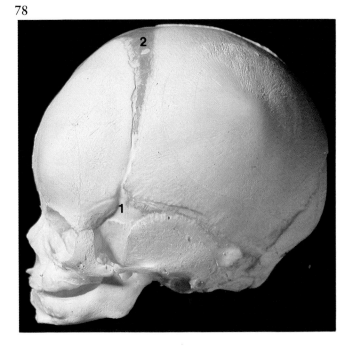

78 The fontanelles. The fontanelles of the skull may be an indication of age in that the anterior fontanelle is said to close by about one and a half years of age, the posterior and anterolateral fontanelles by about three months, and the posterolateral by about one year. These dates are somewhat imprecise for particular individuals.

In this skull the anterolateral fontanelle (1) is still open, indicating that the skull is less than three months after birth. The large anterior fontanelle (2) between the frontal and parietal bones closes at about 18 months of age. This structure may be readily seen on radiographs which provide a non-invasive method of determining approximate age.

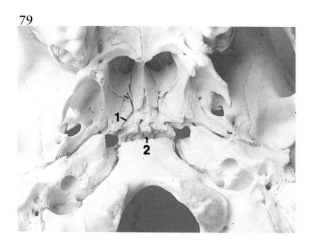

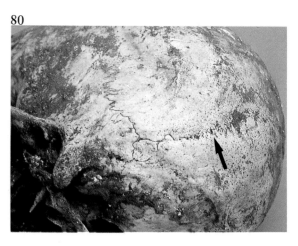

79 Skull cartilages. Bones developing in cartilage can be used to age a skull. At the base of the skull the lateral sphenoidal synchondroses (1) are said to fuse within the first year of life, but the spheno-occipital synchondrosis (2), lying between the basal part of the occipital bone and the adjacent body of the sphenoid, is a major growth centre until later life. In skeletonized material the cartilage itself is lost but radiographs will show whether ossification has occurred. Growth at this site producing an anteroposterior lengthening of the skull base is thought to be associated with the downward and forward movement of the upper face, a process which is necessary to provide sufficient room for the development of the adult dentition. The eruption of the upper second molars occurs at around the age of 12 or 13 years. The spheno-occipital synchondrosis begins to fuse shortly after this, probably slightly earlier in girls than in boys. It provides one of the most useful skeletal ageing factors at this period of development.

80 Skull sutures. Once the end of the second decade has been reached there is relatively little change in the skull, but in later life the sutures between the cranial bones are obliterated, usually from the inside of the cranium outwards. This process begins in the third and fourth decades of life and the sutures may in some cases be completely obliterated in old age. The rate of closure of the sutures varies markedly from individual to individual, and there are examples in the literature of patent sutures in a skull known to be 100 years old at death, whereas in another reported case the sutures had begun to fuse in a 22-year-old. In this case the lambdoid suture, although patent externally (arrow) was in the process of obliteration on its inner aspect, suggesting an age at death of 30 to 55 years.

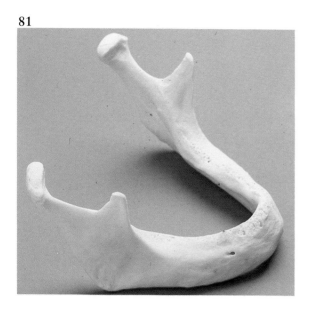

81 Edentulous jaws. In ancient and in some contemporary civilizations where the intervention of a dental surgeon is rare or non-existent, the finding of a completely edentulous mandible indicates an older age group. There will be considerable resorption of the alveolar bone concomitant with a decrease in the major muscle attachment areas of the mandible. The loss of teeth resulting in these changes may be accelerated by pathological changes such as caries or periodontal disease. In so-called advanced societies, patients may be rendered edentulous even in their second or third decades of life by the intervention of their dental surgeon, and regressive changes in the mandible or maxilla may then be accelerated or modified by the provision of full dentures.

Determination of sex

In forensic investigation of skeletal remains the sex should be determined as early as possible, as this will immediately reduce by 50 per cent the number of possible identifications. If the whole skeleton is available the accuracy of sex determination may be of the order of 98 per cent, the pelvic bones alone being the most useful and providing accuracy of around 95 per cent. If only long bones are available accuracy may be reduced to about 80 per cent. There can be no absolute certainty in sex determination, but if all of the features examined tend towards maleness then this would be a reasonable assumption.

82   Shape of the skull. In general, the skull of the male is larger than that of the female, which is more rounded and delicately sculptured. In the male skull (1) the orbits are more square, the nasal apertures higher and narrower with sharper margins. The forehead of the female (2) is usually more vertical but the supraorbital ridges are minimal in size and may be much more rounded than in the male.

82

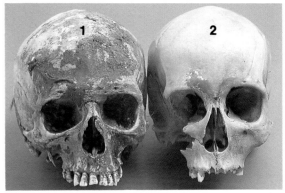

83   Mandibular angle. In the male some investigators have claimed to be able to determine sex with an accuracy of about 90 per cent from the bones of the skull. This is done by studying a number of morphological traits based on the fact that the male skull is frequently more muscularly developed than that of the female. The lateral aspect of the angle of the mandible in the male frequently shows a marked roughening or ridged appearance due to the attachment of the masseter muscles, the powerful closing muscles of the jaw. The lower border of the angle (arrow) may deviate laterally to a marked extent in the male.

83

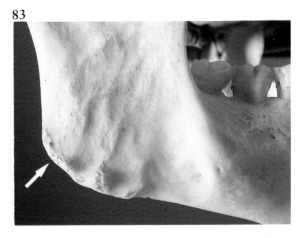

84   Female mandible. In the female, the angle of the jaw is often more rounded and gracile in construction, and the attachment surface for the masseter muscle (1) is frequently much smoother. These features will, in general, only be obvious well after puberty when secondary sexual characteristics have developed. Even then, no single feature on the skull may in itself be sufficient for sex determination to be made. A muscular female may show many characteristics of the male, and the reverse may often be the case.

84

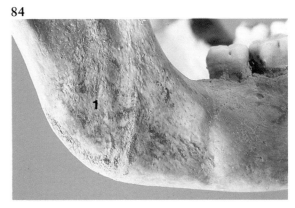

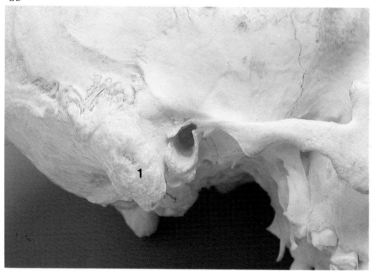

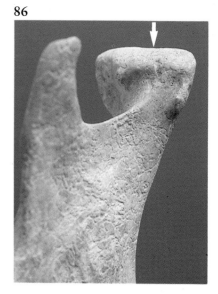

85 Mastoid process. This structure would be expected to be larger, more prominent and more roughened in the male than in the female. In this example, the mastoid process (1), which is just behind the ear canal, is elongated and has a pitted and roughened surface: these features indicate maleness. The female mastoid process would be expected to be modelled more delicately and have a smoother surface for attachment of muscle. Other features indicative of a male skull are larger occipital condyles, a larger and broader U-shaped palate, and heavier and more laterally arched cheek bones.

86 Condylar head. The complex joint between the lower jaw and the skull is made up of a 'socket' in the skull base and a rounded head on the mandible known as the condyle (arrow). In some populations certain measurements of this structure may vary sufficiently between male and female skulls to make this a useful method of determining sex.

Determination of race

Although in modern times there has been much interbreeding, thus lessening the differences between them, most of mankind can be grouped into negroid, caucasoid and mongoloid races. Because of the intermixing of hereditary characteristics, people may be classified sociologically as belonging to various clear cut races, whereas biologically they may be a mixture of many.

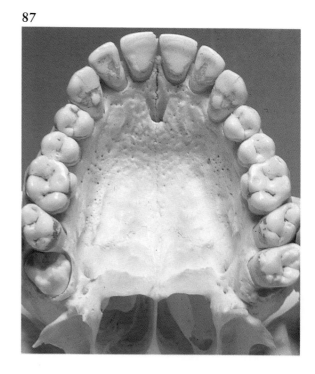

87 Facial features. The facial features of the living are reflected in the underlying skeletal structures, so that the nasal aperture of the negroid skull may be broad, and mongoloid skulls may have larger prominent cheekbones. Racial differences are less marked in the female, so that the biggest variation between two adjacent skulls would be expected to be found between a male negroid on the one hand and a female caucasoid on the other. This example is a negroid palate, which is U-shaped and broad with protruding anterior teeth.

Missing teeth

When the jaw bones are examined it is important to determine whether teeth missing from the arch have been lost ante-mortem and if so, how long before death.

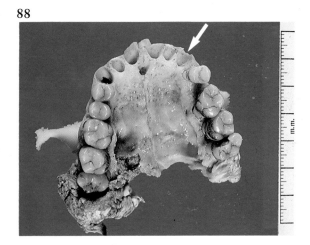

88 Post-mortem loss. If the tooth is lost after death, either as a result of decomposition of the body or scavenging by animals, the bone surrounding the socket will not have reacted to the loss of the tooth and the margins of the socket would be unresorbed and have a sharp profile. If a tooth is lost a matter of a few days before death it may be difficult to determine the exact chronology of the event from an examination of the bone. In this example, the sharp margins of the sockets of the front teeth (arrow) indicate that loss of teeth occurred after death.

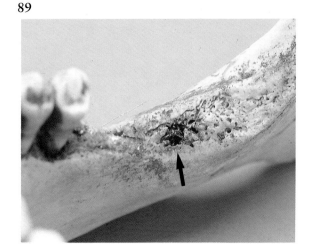

89 Ante-mortem loss. When teeth are removed before death a blood clot forms within the socket and this rapidly organizes into granulation tissue (see **186**). New bone is progressively laid down both on the walls of the socket and within the granulation tissue and the socket will have a granular appearance as the new bone mineralizes. The bone filling the healing socket may have an irregular appearance for some time after the extraction (arrow), and it may be difficult to determine exactly when the tooth was removed. In the first few days following an extraction it may be possible to curette out the remnants of granulation tissue and to determine histologically the stage of healing of the socket. This may be useful where a person is accusing an assailant of having knocked a tooth out at a particular time, and the forensic dentist may confirm this from microscopic examination.

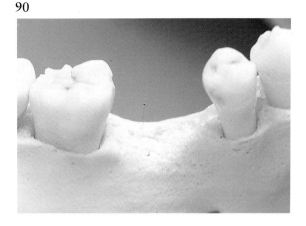

90 Remodelling. As healing of the socket progresses the bone may be completely remodelled so that little or no evidence of the extraction site is left. In this specimen there is still some remodelling occurring on the crest of the alveolar ridge which has resorbed leaving a saddle-like area. Remodelling of a socket is variable, and will depend upon the particular healing characteristics of the individual, their age, the amount of trauma that occurred at the time of extraction, and whether subsequent infection was present. The forensic dentist should be cautious in attributing a particular time-span to the stage of healing, but it is likely that if the alveolar crest has a smooth and cortical surface at least a year will have elapsed since the tooth was removed.

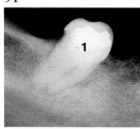

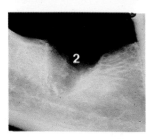

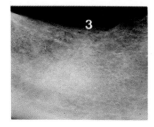

91 Radiographs of healing sockets. Radiographs of healing tooth sockets may give some indication of the length of time that has elapsed since the tooth was lost. The molar tooth (1) was extracted and two months later the outline of the socket (2) is still visible, but the margins are becoming indistinct. Eighteen months after the extraction (3) the socket area has been replaced with new bone.

The rate at which healing progresses and the appearance on radiographs are very variable and should be interpreted with caution.

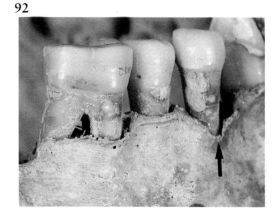

92 Supporting bone loss. In a young person the crests of the bone supporting the teeth usually lie within about 2 mm of the cervical margin of the teeth, so that usually only this length of the root of a tooth is exposed in the young skeleton. As age progresses, inflammation of the junction of the tooth and gum may eventually result in the crest of the alveolar bone (arrow) being resorbed so that more of the root is exposed. Examination of a skull may, therefore, give some indication of disease of the gums during life.

Time since death

If sufficient time has elapsed for skeletonization of the body to occur, it is not possible to be precise in estimating time of death. In these circumstances information should be sought from as many sources as possible.

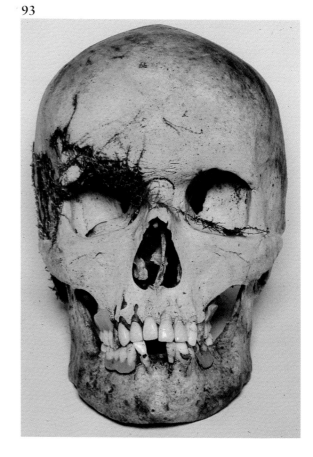

93 Effects of weather. These skeletonized remains were found in a wooded area and it was reported that the Forestry Commission inspected the ground at least every three years, so that the body could not have lain there for longer than that period. The effects of different weathering patterns on a skeleton are well illustrated here as the mandible was buried, whereas the maxilla and cranium were exposed, thus making estimates of time of death even more difficult. Porcelain crowns and partial dentures were present (see **64**) and an analysis of the type of porcelain used to construct these restorations indicated that they were probably made around 1970, as advances in porcelain technology have since rendered them obsolete. Examination of the scene at which the body was found revealed, at some distance, fragments of a jacket pocket containing both decimal and non-decimal coinage, thus confirming the probable time of death as 1971.

Skull radiographs in identification

Some skull features are best examined using radiographs, and these include the sella turcica, air sinuses and the presence of pathological change.

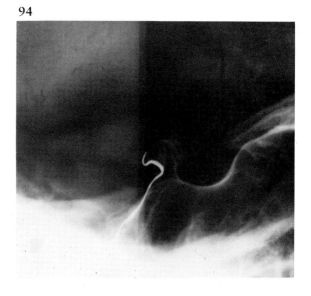

94   Sella turcica. The shape of certain parts of the skull may be individually distinctive. Some authorities believe that the sella turcica, the area of the skull base adjacent to the pituitary gland, is such a feature. However, this shape may change with age and can be affected by the presence of tumours.

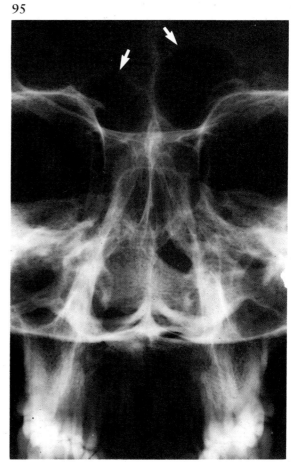

95   Air sinuses. Of all the bony structures in the skull, the air sinuses have probably been most often used in identification procedures. Of these, the frontal sinuses above the inner aspect of the eyes (arrows) are said to be most reliable. Classifications have included their shape, deviation of the septum between the sinuses, characteristics of the upper border, presence or absence of partial septae, and extensions into the adjacent bone. The shape of the adult frontal sinuses may remain unchanged throughout life, and it is said that even identical twins have different shaped sinuses.

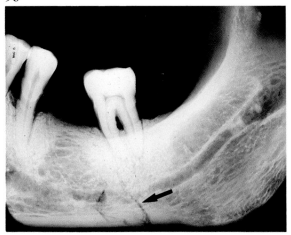

96 Previous bone pathology. A wide range of diseases may affect and modify the structure of the skeleton during life. These may be broadly classified as trauma, infections, tumours, endocrine disorders, nutritional disturbances and developmental deformities. Fractures through the mandible or maxilla may be visible on radiographs, as in this example (arrow). There is no evidence of healing or of callus formation so that the trauma probably took place at or around the time of death. It is important to screen the skull for the presence of fractures, especially in cases of possible child abuse. Post-mortem damage may occur to the bones of the skull resulting in fractures from earth pressure, from animal damage or from careless excavation. It is usually possible, by examining the margins of the fracture, to determine under what circumstances it occurred.

Surgical artefacts

97

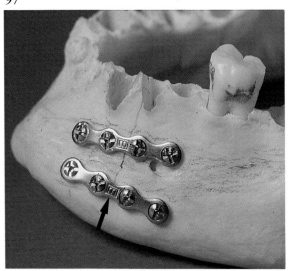

97 Bone plates. Positive identification from bones alone is not usually possible, so in cases where there are no distinctive dental features, or dental records are unavailable, identification may never be made. After trauma, in unfavourable or comminuted fractures with displacement the fracture ends may be reduced by the insertion of pins on either side of the fracture line. These are removed postoperatively and may eventually leave no permanent record in the bone. In other cases lower border wires may be inserted, and likewise, providing death has not occurred within a few weeks of the operation, would normally be removed leaving no permanent mark. In other cases bone plates may be screwed across the fracture line and these are frequently left in situ as long as they present no problem to the patient. In these instances the type of bone plate used and in some cases an inscribed maker's name or number (arrow) may enable identification to be followed through.

Chapter 7
The soft tissues

The mainstay of dental identification is comparison of the post-mortem findings of the teeth and fillings with ante-mortem records. However, it is important that examination of the soft tissues should not be ignored.

By contrast with the hard tissues, which are relatively inert, the soft tissues alter in response to local environmental conditions and are also subject to a wide range of diseases. Recognition of the changes may contribute to identification by highlighting such factors as habits or responses to particular drugs. Pigmentation of the oral soft tissues may give a useful indication of race.

Two particular aspects of distinctive soft tissue characteristics have been suggested as potentially valuable for identification. These are the lines in the lips—the lip print—and the pattern of the rugae or ridges present on the front part of the roof of the mouth.

Soft tissue pigmentation

98

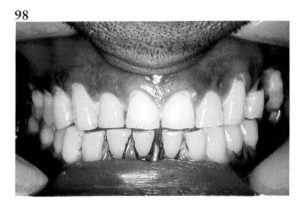

98 Racial pigmentation. Pigmentation in the oral mucosa, particularly the gums, is roughly proportional to skin pigmentation. The pigment is melanin, the same pigment that is present in skin. This can be particularly useful in suggesting the race of an individual when the body is so severely burned that no skin remains.

99

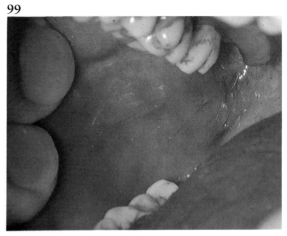

99 Pigmentation caused by dietary habits. The yellowish pigmentation of the cheek in this individual is caused by eating curry over a long period. This case was unusual in that the individual was a white woman who had married an Indian man and adopted his dietary habits. Such characteristic features of oral soft tissues may be preserved surprisingly well even when the body is badly burned.

Mucosal disease

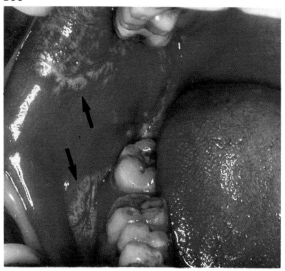

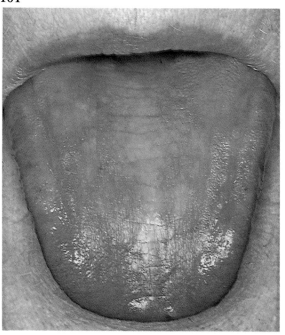

100 Mucosal disease. This man was suffering from a disease of the soft tissues which has given rise to slightly elevated white striae in parts of his cheeks (arrows). This is a lichenoid reaction which has an unusual distribution for such an abnormality. It was caused by a food allergy to dietary spices. This abnormality was painful and is the type of distinctive detail which would be recalled by the family of this man.

101 Tongue features. Physicians have traditionally examined the tongue for evidence of ill-health. The woman illustrated has a smooth tongue which seems covered by an unusually thin surface layer of epithelium. This is characteristic of nutritional deficiency such as iron or some vitamins. There are various reasons for such deficiency. One example is chronic alcoholism.

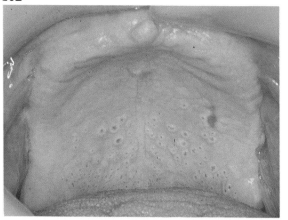

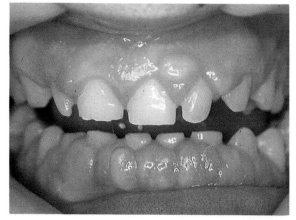

102 Soft tissue changes related to smoking. It is sometimes possible to detect evidence of habits because of changes in the soft tissues. This elderly man smoked a pipe and did not wear his denture. The smoking has caused an overall whiteness of the palate resulting from hyperkeratosis, with small red areas which are the orifices of the ducts of minor salivary glands.

103 Drug-induced soft tissue changes. The gums in this adolescent show considerable overgrowth, almost covering the lower teeth. This is a side-effect of phenytoin, one of the drugs used in the treatment of epilepsy. A less frequent cause of the same type of overgrowth is cyclosporin, a drug given to transplant patients to prevent graft rejection.

Lip prints

The red part of the lips is known as the vermilion border. The lines and grooves present on this area are said to be characteristic for each individual and to remain the same throughout life. In this respect they are analagous to fingerprints. The possibility of using lip prints for identification arises particularly in females using lipstick, where marks from kissing or the lips being pressed against a tissue or a handkerchief may provide a record of the lip print. This is a very infrequent form of forensic odontological identification which has been mainly described in Japan, but it is a possibility that should not be forgotten.

104 Lip details. Although this woman's lips are large, the details of the individual lip lines are not particularly well marked. The grooves form a mixture of patterns, some being straight, some intersecting and in the lower lip some form a fine network pattern.

104

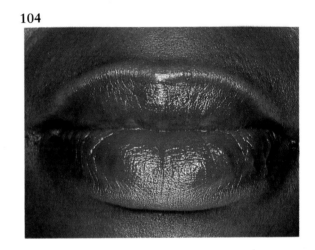

105

105 Lip print. This print was made by the woman shown in **104** in the manner of someone using a napkin or a handkerchief to blot the lips. This only records a print if the individual is wearing lipstick. It is a poor print, recording only parts of the lips. It is clearly identifiable as a lip print and it is possible to see some correspondence between the patterns of lines. Many experts are hesitant to identify from lip prints and it is doubtful if the woman in **104** could be identified from this print.

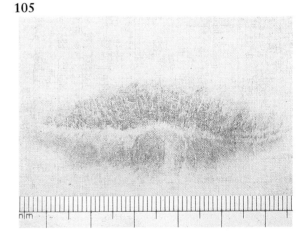

106

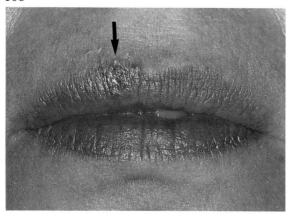

106 Lip details. This woman has distinct lip lines which form well-marked grooves, most of which are straight and run the full width of the vermilion border. An area of abnormality is present, caused by a cold sore which has almost healed (arrow).

107

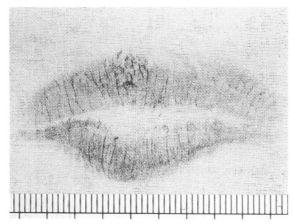

107 Lip print. This is a mirror image view so that it can be compared directly with the view of the lips in **106**. The area of irregular patterns caused by the cold sore is obvious, but in addition there is clear correspondence between the patterns of other areas of the lip lines, and a positive identification of this woman could be made from this lip print.

Palatal rugae

The pattern of the rugae or ridges at the front of the roof of the mouth is said to be characteristic of each individual. These may be altered following the loss of teeth.

108

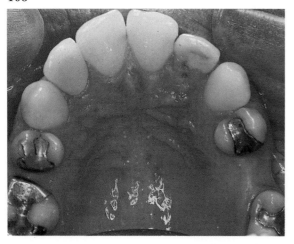

108 Palatal rugae. The ridges on the front of the roof of the mouth are clearly shown in this view. The difficulty of using these for identification purposes is that sources of records with details of palatal rugae are likely to be available in very few instances where identification is required. The possibilities would include intra-oral photographs in dental or medical records, dental casts or old dentures.

Soft tissue tattoos

Inadvertent tattoos of oral mucosa sometimes occur when fragments of amalgam filling material become lodged in the tissues. Much less frequently, deliberate tattooing of the soft tissues of the mouth, particularly the inner aspect of the lip may be encountered.

109

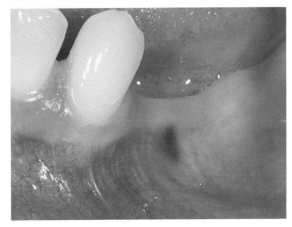

109 Amalgam tattoo. The discrete blue-grey pigmentation in this patient could be caused by an uncommon form of endogenous melanin-containing lesion, but is much more likely to be exogenous pigmentation caused by amalgam. The amalgam is derived from filling material that has become lodged in the soft tissues, usually of the cheek or lips. It is a distinctive feature which is likely to be recorded in a patient's records. It may also be evident on radiographs.

110

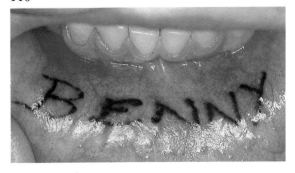

110 Tattoo on lips. An unusual case of identification was made from this tattoo inside the lower lip. Tattooing of this nature is a rather painful and uncommon event and it may be assumed that an individual would submit to such a procedure only if it had some particular significance. It has been suggested that this form of tattooing is seen in some homosexuals and in drug pushers.

Soft tissue injuries

111

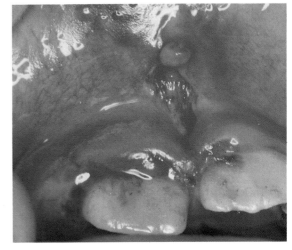

111 Non-accidental injuries. The mouth may show evidence of trauma, such as the ruptured fraenum in this upper lip. This type of injury may be seen in cases of non-accidental injury to children and it is important that the forensic dentist should note such features in addition to identification evidence.

Chapter 8
Age determination from the teeth

The ageing of unknown human remains is based upon a detailed knowledge of biological changes that occur during development, growth and maturation. The exact chronology of these changes is dependent upon physiological variations in any one individual, and studies produce at best an estimate of age which may not correspond to the true calendar age of the person concerned. Many techniques are based upon post-cranial parts of the anatomy not directly related to the facial structures, and these lie outside the scope of this text. Details of these methods may be found in the relevant literature. This chapter is confined to approaches within the expertise of the forensic odontologist. It is convenient to look at the problem from four standpoints: changes occurring during fetal life, those associated with the period around birth, those from birth to the onset of the third decade and those from young adulthood to old age.

Prenatal development

The forensic dentist is rarely involved in the ageing of the unborn fetus, but occasionally premature births or abortion specimens may have to be aged.

112

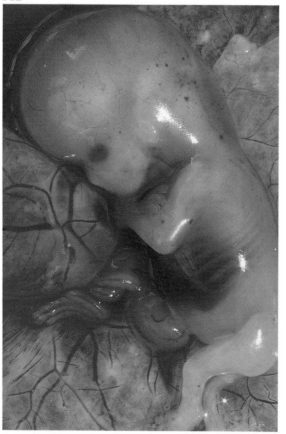

112 The human fetus. The first signs of tooth development in man are seen at about six weeks of intra-uterine life when the downgrowths of the oral epithelium (the dental laminae) develop. Individual tooth germs differentiate at the future sites of the deciduous teeth, and later the permanent molars, but it is not until about 16 weeks that the first of these, the deciduous incisors, begin to mineralize. This fetus was about nine weeks at death so tooth germ development would be well advanced. Before this important stage the position of the germs may be visible as radiolucent areas on radiographs, but detailed examination of them is possible only by taking histological sections through the jaw. The chronology of cellular differentiation in the different tooth germs may be found in standard texts of dental anatomy.

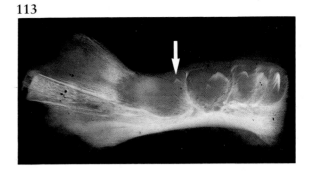

113 Jaw of twenty-six week fetus. In this radiograph of the mandible of an unborn human fetus some of the tooth germs have begun to mineralize. The process is well advanced in the anterior teeth, and in the crypt for the first deciduous molar the mineralized outline of two cusps can be seen. In the crypt for the second deciduous molar (arrow) initial mineralization of one cusp is just visible, and as this process starts at about six months of intra-uterine life this child was about 26 weeks from conception at the time of death. Posterior to the crypt for the second deciduous molar is the early formation of the crypt for the first permanent molar. No evidence of mineralization is seen in this tooth at this stage. Fetal skeletons may also be aged from the lengths of certain of the long bones and the mandible, and tables of expected dimensions are available.

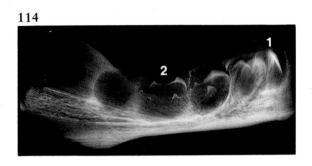

114 Jaw of thirty week fetus. Mineralization of the anterior teeth is now more obvious and the crown in the incisor region (1) on the right of the picture is about three-fifths complete. The crypt of the lower second deciduous molar (2) contains a tooth with five cusps which are beginning to mineralize, but they are widely separated. In the first deciduous molar, the cusps have begun to fuse together but are still not completely united. There is no evidence of mineralization in the first permanent molar. These features indicate that this fetus has not yet reached full term and is probably about 30 weeks from conception.

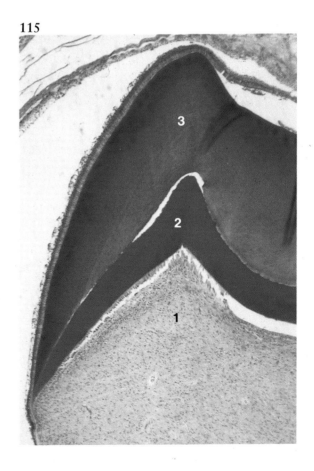

115 Histology. Standard radiographs of fetal material may sometimes be difficult to interpret because the extent of mineralization may not be clearly seen. Ageing may be confirmed from sections through the jaw and tooth so that the stage of hard tissue formation may be studied. In this section through a molar tooth the papilla can be seen (1) and above it the mineralizing dentine (2). The enamel matrix (3) is not yet mature and has not been lost during the demineralization procedure. Active ameloblasts are present at the periphery of the enamel matrix indicating that the outline of the crown is not yet complete. As this section is of the mesiolingual cusp of a deciduous lower molar, the age at death is probably about eight months from conception. Because the organic component in the enamel decreases during maturation, another method of ageing the fetus and newborn is to estimate biochemically the amount of organic material present and to relate this information to developing teeth of known maturity.

Age determination in the newborn

During birth the fetal skull has to be compressed so that it can pass down the birth canal. This is possible because the bones of the vault are spaced out with connective tissue which forms the fontanelles (see 78). These are replaced by bone in the period after birth so that the sutures are formed.

116

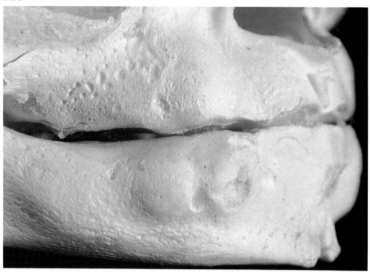

116 Jaws of the newborn child. The absence of erupted teeth in the normal child suggests that the age is less than six months, but eruption times are notoriously variable. It is not unknown for teeth (usually lower incisors) to be erupted at birth, and these are referred to as neonatal teeth. The orbits are relatively well developed at this stage, whilst the jaws are of minimum bone height as they are not yet required to support erupted teeth. The brain and hence the cranial vault are proportionally large so that the face of the newborn appears to be diminutive when compared with the total size of the baby's head.

117

117 Radiograph of mandible. This radiograph of the lower jaw at birth shows several features which are useful in age estimation. The cusps of the first deciduous molar have mineralized and have fused producing a continuous occlusal surface (1). In the second deciduous molar some of the cusps have fused but there is still no continuity across the whole of the occlusal surface. Within the crypt of the first permanent molar one of the mesial cusps has started to mineralize (arrow) indicating a newborn infant.

Stillborn infants

It is frequently important for medicolegal reasons to determine whether the body of an infant is that of a newborn or a stillborn child. If the soft tissues are reasonably intact it may be possible, from the changes occurring at birth in the lungs, heart and surrounding vessels, to determine whether the child actually had an independent existence. If the soft tissues have been destroyed and only skeletal material is available, this may be much more difficult.

118

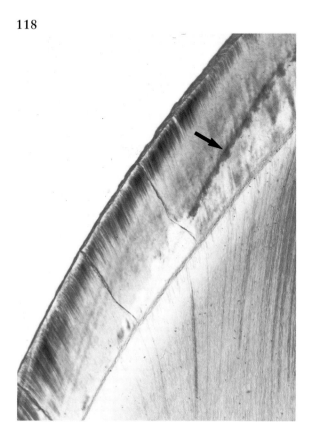

118 Neonatal line. Some of the teeth begin their development before birth and growth continues through birth into the neonatal period. When the child is born the physiological upset results in a change in metabolic activity of the cells producing the hard tissues of the tooth. An accentuated growth or incremental line frequently results, in both the enamel and the dentine. In this microscopic ground section of the deciduous tooth of a child, such an accentuated incremental line can be seen in the outer enamel dividing the prenatal enamel nearest to the dentine from the postnatal enamel nearest to the surface of the tooth (arrow). For such a neonatal line to be clearly visible with the light microscope, a reasonable thickness of postnatal enamel has to be produced. In practice, this means that the method can be used only if the child survives for about three weeks after birth.

119

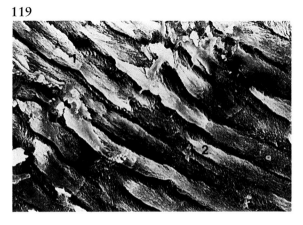

119 Scanning electron microscopy. The difficulty of resolving the neonatal line microscopically can be overcome by searching for it with the scanning electron microscope. This instrument allows for much higher resolution than the light microscope and the individual rods or prisms making up the structure of enamel can easily be seen, although they are no more than 5 μm in diameter. At the time of birth there is sufficient disturbance to produce structural changes in these rods. These changes may be a disturbance in crystal growth, a change in direction of the rods, or an alteration in their dimension. The rods are laid down at a rate of approximately 4 μm per day so it should be possible to distinguish postnatal enamel (1) from prenatal enamel (2) within a day or two of birth.

Age determination during the first two decades of life

During the first six months of life no teeth are clinically visible in the baby's mouth, but this does not mean that changes are not occurring within the jaws.

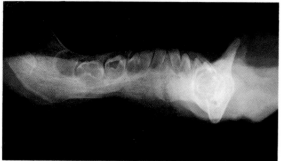

120 Radiography. A child's body was exhumed by a dog walking with its owner. Considerable putrefaction had taken place. Non-invasive radiographs were taken before any tissues were removed. This radiograph of the mandible suggests that the deciduous incisor crowns are now complete (1) and the crown of the first molar is well on its way to completion (2). The occlusal surface of the second deciduous molar is continuous, and there is a mineralized cusp tip visible in the mesial part of the first permanent molar (arrow). This degree of development of the dentition would indicate an age of around three months after birth.

121

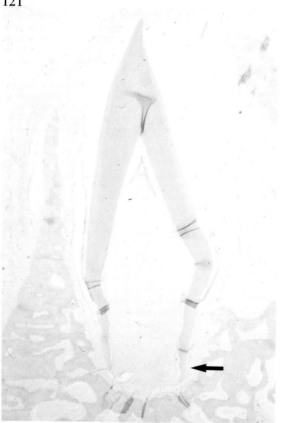

121 Histological studies. This section was taken from the same body as in **120**, and even when considerable putrefaction has taken place and staining is difficult, the cell outlines in the pulp, periodontal ligament and bone marrow spaces can still be seen. Ageing of an unknown body from the dentition is done first by using the eruption status of the teeth, and second by studying the degree of their development. This tooth is the lower central incisor and the degree of root development (arrow) confirms the age of three months after birth.

122 Eruption sequence. This child's body had been immersed in water for some weeks after death and it would not be appropriate to seek identification from visual facial features. Age estimation would be possible using radiographs of the long bones and epiphyses, but may also be confirmed by an examination of the dentition. Visual examination of the erupted teeth showed that the deciduous dentition was complete and therefore the child would be expected to be at least two and a half years of age. However, there was as yet no evidence of eruption of the first permanent molar. A radiograph of the mandible confirmed the status of the deciduous dentition and also confirmed that the first permanent molar was just in position to erupt. The estimated age of just less than six years was entirely compatible with the known age of a missing child.

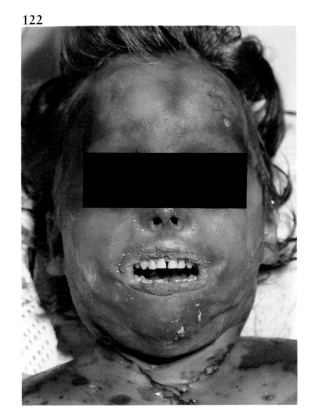

123 Permanent teeth. The first permanent teeth to erupt into the oral cavity and come into full occlusion are the first molars (1). They are followed about six months to a year later by the eruption of first the lower and then the upper central incisors. In this skull the permanent upper central incisors have not yet reached the occlusal plane (2). The deciduous lateral incisors, canines and molars are still present and the age would be around seven years. A radiograph of the molar region showed the presence of a developing second permanent molar, the crown of which was virtually complete, confirming the age of seven to eight years.

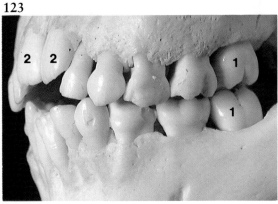

124 Root resorption in the mixed dentition. The stage where both deciduous and permanent teeth are present together is known as the mixed dentition stage. As time progresses the deciduous teeth will resorb and be exfoliated, thus allowing the permanent teeth below them to erupt into occlusion. The degree of resorption of the root of the deciduous tooth (arrow) may therefore be a useful age indicator. Variations in resorption of the deciduous teeth occur depending upon the presence or absence of their permanent successors. It is important that the whole dentition be examined in detail so that ageing is based on as many features as possible.

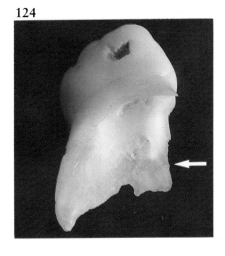

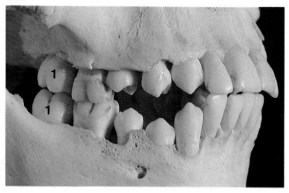

125 Teenage dentition. In this skeleton the second molars (1) have erupted into occlusion and the premolars are erupting and reaching their functional position. The degree of accuracy of ageing becomes less in older individuals, and from an examination of clinically visible teeth it would only be possible to age this skull at somewhere between 10 and 13 years. As in previous examples, it is advisable to take radiographs so that the position and degree of development of all the teeth including their roots can be ascertained.

126

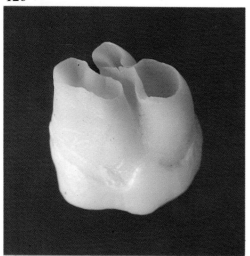

126 The wisdom teeth. Although the timing of eruption of the wisdom teeth may be variable, the process of development of the roots is a more reliable guide to age. When a tooth erupts, the root is about two-thirds complete, and it has been shown that the root apices are always complete at around age 23 to 24 years. In this example the roots are approximately half formed, indicating that the individual was around 17 years of age. The completion of the apices of the third molar mark the point after which age estimation from development and eruption of the teeth is no longer a useful method.

127

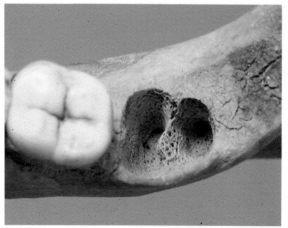

127 Tooth sockets. An unknown body may be aged from the stages of development and eruption of the teeth, but there may also be evidence of the stage of tooth development in the skeleton even when the teeth are not present. In this case the mandible of a young adult was found separated from the remainder of the body and the lower third molar had been lost. Examination of the base of the socket of the two roots shows that there are flattened areas of bone suggesting that the third molar tooth had not completed its development. This fragment was aged from this feature alone as belonging to a person of approximately 22 years.

Age determination after the first two decades of life

Once the development of crowns and roots is completed and the teeth are in functional occlusion, age determination using dental findings becomes more difficult. However, ageing by long bone criteria or closure of sutures and synchondroses is also subject to variation so dental estimates of age are still extremely useful in forensic investigations. After the age of about 24 years dental estimates depend upon subtle changes in the teeth which are dependent not only upon increasing age but also upon the effects of wear and tear.

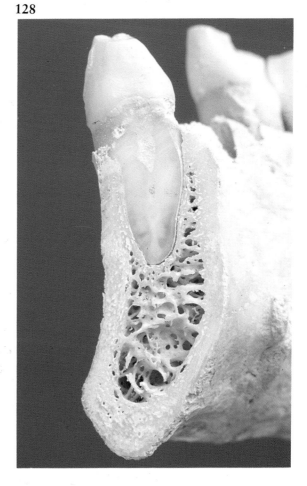

128 Translucent apices. Skeletons older than 24 years at death become increasingly difficult to age and usually require preparation of sections through the teeth (see **129**). If such specialized techniques are not available, useful information may be obtained by cutting through the mandible or maxilla alongside a standing permanent tooth. In this case the mandible has been sectioned immediately next to the distal surface of a lower canine. The root of the tooth is not uniformly opaque throughout its length, there being a degree of translucency near to the apex. This change is related to age rather than to pathology in the tooth. The apical translucency is minimal or absent in a 20-year-old but involves at least half of the root of the tooth in someone aged 70 years.

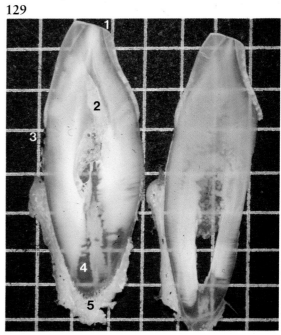

129 Age determination using tooth sections. Gustafson described a method for ageing the dead which was based upon changes occurring in the teeth as age progresses. He awarded arbitrary points to the degree of occlusal wear (1), the amount of secondary dentine in the pulp chamber (2), the level of the gum attachment around the neck of the tooth (3), the extent of translucent or sclerotic apical dentine (4), the amount of secondary cementum at the apex (5) and the extent of resorption of the apex. This latter feature has been shown to be very unreliable and is no longer used.

If any of these features is unchanged from the situation in a tooth which has recently completed its development then no points are awarded. Minimal change, for example enamel wear but not extending to dentine is awarded one point. Severe change, for example translucency extending halfway up the root, is awarded three points. The points awarded to each feature are added and the total compared with a regression line prepared from teeth of known age. The method requires considerable expertise and should be attempted only by a dentist practised in its use.

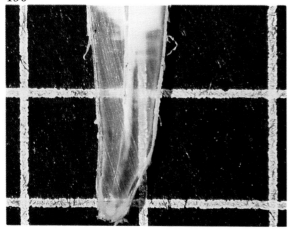

130 Translucent apical dentine. The most reliable change in ageing teeth appears to be the extent of sclerotic or translucent apical dentine. Various methods have been suggested to quantify this phenomenon, one of them uses sections through the teeth 1 mm in thickness and another uses accurate measurement of the translucent area rather than awarding points based on its extent. This latter method used alone on one tooth is said to be capable of estimating age to within five years in about 60 per cent of cases. However, further studies of this technique are necessary because it has recently been shown that the translucent zone is not symmetrical in the root apex, so the determined age may depend upon the direction in which the tooth is sectioned.

Chapter 9
Full dentures

The term 'full denture' is used when no teeth remain in the upper or lower jaw and the denture replaces all the teeth of that jaw. Several identification techniques can be used with full dentures. Occasionally the name of the patient is marked on the appliance. Not infrequently, laboratory marks are included which may indicate the first letter of the surname of the owner or give other information about the laboratory in which the denture was made.

It is sometimes necessary to be able to relate one denture to the opposed denture with which it has been worn. This is most readily accomplished when they have been worn as a set for a considerable period.

When teeth are extracted progressive changes occur in the mouth over a long period. There is reduction in the size of the jaw bones upon which dentures rest. This means that when an individual appliance is worn for a long time it becomes gradually looser. This may make it difficult to state that a denture definitely does fit an individual jaw, although it is often easy to say that a particular denture could not fit.

Analysis of the materials used in the construction of dentures can sometimes be of value in identification. However, a relatively limited range of materials is used and this can pose difficulties. In the great majority of cases the pink material used as the denture base is acrylic. The teeth are usually acrylic, but may be porcelain. A range of tooth shapes and shades is available. If the dentist's records give details of the tooth mould and shade used for an individual patient, this may assist in identification. It is unlikely that identification could be accomplished by examination of the denture base and tooth materials alone.

Construction of full dentures

131

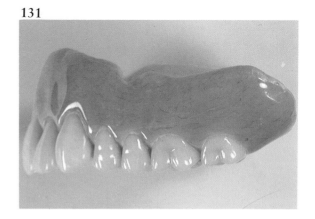

131 Denture base material. Acrylic is the material most frequently used for denture bases. A small range of shades is available and some also have 'veining' from the inclusion of fine coloured nylon threads. This makes the denture base appear more lifelike. Newer denture base materials such as nylon are being investigated, but these are not in general use.

132

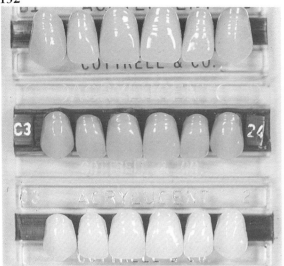

132 Tooth mould and shape. A range of artificial teeth is available in both acrylic and porcelain. The dentist will prescribe the teeth to be used by the technician for a given patient. If this detail is noted in the dentist's record it can assist in identification.

133

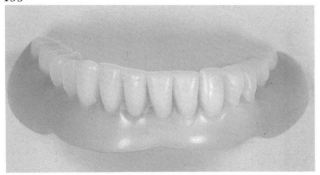

133 Variation in workmanship. This lower denture has been constructed in acrylic, with acrylic teeth. The technical work in the setting up of the teeth and in the finish of the denture base is crude. This is a denture which is likely to have been made as inexpensively as possible.

134

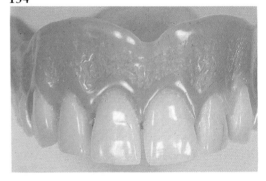

134 Variation in workmanship. This denture contrasts sharply with that shown in **133** as it shows a much better quality of workmanship. The denture base has been carefully fashioned to make it appear more lifelike. The teeth are a better shape and have been set up to give a pleasing distinctive appearance. This type of denture is likely to have been made in a high quality laboratory.

135

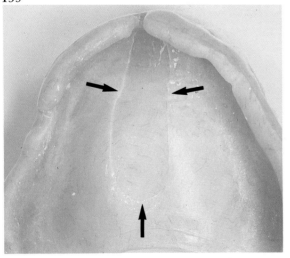

135 Variables in denture construction. This is the palatal surface of an upper denture. The area indicated by the arrows is a palatal relief area: the denture has been constructed with a shallow recess to prevent it pressing too hard on the midline of the palate where the bone is covered by only a thin layer of soft tissue. The shapes of palatal relief areas used by individual technicians are quite variable and may allow a dentist or a dental technician to recognize his or her own work.

Marks and names in dentures

The marks in dentures which most frequently aid identification are those made in the production laboratory to ensure that work for different patients is not confused. This may be a name, but is more often just an initial. Dentures may also be marked as a deliberate policy to enable the identity of the owner to be determined. From time to time it has been advocated that either the patient's name or some other identifiable mark, such as the National Insurance number should be incorporated in the denture. For reasons of cost it is unlikely that such naming of dentures will be undertaken routinely in the UK.

136

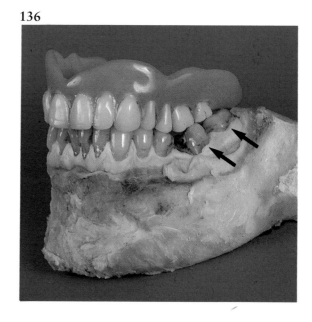

136 Acrylic denture. The man whose teeth are illustrated died on a bus. No evidence of identity was present on the body. Dental examination revealed that he wore a full upper denture opposed to his own natural teeth. The denture base material is acrylic and the teeth are also acrylic. They have been set in a slightly unusual arrangement to allow for the tilted position of the lower left molar teeth against which the denture bites (arrows).

137

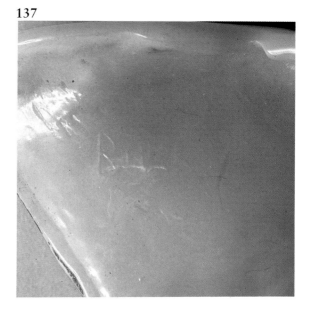

137 Name in denture. When the denture shown in **136** was examined carefully, it was apparent that a name, although not easy to see, was present on the fitting surface. The name is Bally and this enabled the police to identify the man from the voters' register of the district to which the bus was travelling. In this case the patient's name had been marked on the model of the upper jaw which had been used for the construction of the denture. It is probable that this had been done by the technician in order to avoid mixing up work from different patients.

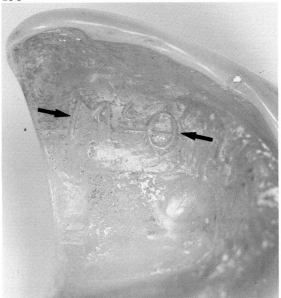

138 Marks in dentures. Names are infrequently found in dentures, but it is not uncommon to see laboratory marks. Often only one letter is present, and if this is so, the letter is likely to be the first letter of the surname of the patient. In the denture illustrated the letters McO (arrows) were present on the fitting surface of the upper denture. This came from an unidentified body recovered in poor condition from a river. The presence of the marks in the denture allowed the body to be fairly quickly identified as a missing person with the unusual surname of McOliphant.

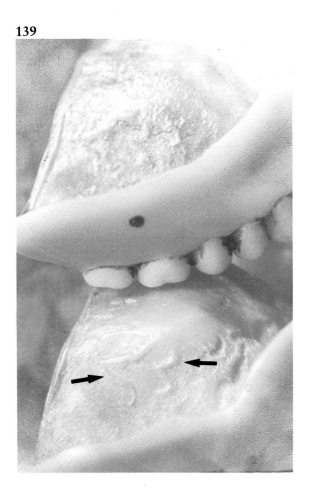

139 Marks in dentures. The illustration is of an unusual case where identification of a body was accomplished from marks in the denture. The view shows parts of two upper dentures made for the same patient. The uppermost denture was with the body at the time of death. The other denture had been made several years previously and was found in the man's home. On the fitting surface of the older denture there is a laboratory mark which is an inverted number 23 (arrows). This number had been scratched on the model of the upper jaw and therefore appeared in relief on the fitting surface of the denture. When worn over a period of time this had caused an indentation in the roof of the mouth. This had subsequently been transferred to the impression taken for the construction of the new dentures and was evident on the fitting surface of the denture found on the body.

140 Permanent marking of dentures. Acrylic dentures are made by constructing a mould into which the denture base material is packed whilst of a 'doughy' consistency before being polymerized to the final hard plastic. A name on tissue paper can be incorporated into the denture at the mould stage. Alternatively, as in the denture illustrated, a small recess can be prepared in the finished denture to allow a name to be inserted. The recess can then be filled with self-curing acrylic. If desired, the name can be made less conspicuous by placing it on the fitting surface of the denture.

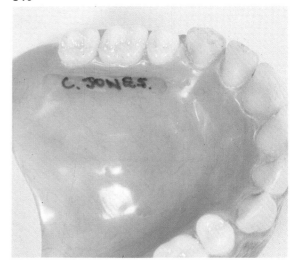

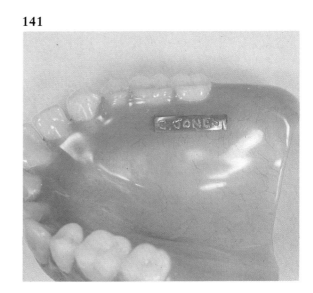

141 Permanent marking of dentures. The label with the patient's name or identifying mark can be made in a number of ways. An alternative to the paper used in **140** is for the name to be inscribed on a thin metal strip and incorporated into the denture. One possible advantage of this would be that the name or mark would be less likely to be destroyed if the denture was burned.

142 Short-term marking of dentures. In a hospital ward with many elderly patients wearing dentures, problems can arise for staff and patients in ensuring correct identification of dentures. One simple practical method of marking dentures in this situation is for a part of the denture base to be roughened, for example with fine sandpaper, to provide a suitable surface upon which the patient's name can be written in ink or ball-point pen. The name can then be sealed with a layer of clear nail varnish.

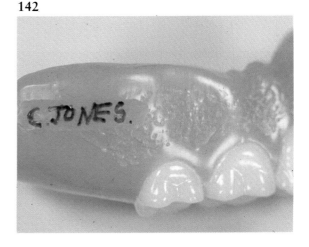

Matching of upper and lower dentures

For each individual patient, upper and lower dentures are constructed with care to ensure that they bite against each other evenly. After a period of use, corresponding patterns of wear will develop in opposed teeth and these can assist in relating a denture to its 'mate' as illustrated in the following case.

143

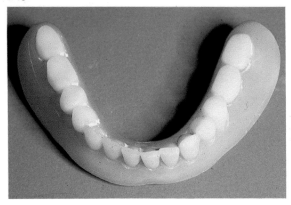

143 Denture at scene of crime. This case involved a drunken man who pushed aside a young man who was trying to help him to his feet. The young man tripped, hit his head on the pavement and subsequently died. The drunken man then staggered away. This acrylic lower denture was found at the scene and the problem was to determine whether or not this lower denture belonged to the drunken man. The standard of workmanship is poor, and the amount of wear on the teeth, particularly the back teeth, is very considerable, suggesting that the denture has been worn for a long time. It was possible to fit the lower denture to the lower jaw of the accused man. However, it fitted loosely, which was not surprising in view of the period of time the denture was likely to have been in use.

144

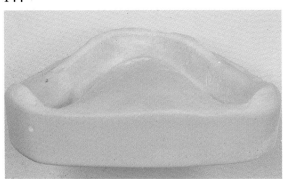

144 Model from a denture. Visual confirmation of the similarity of the denture to the jaw was obtained by preparing a model from the fitting surface of the denture and comparing this with a model of the lower jaw of the accused man. This model was cast from the fitting surface of the denture shown in **143**. It shows the view looking at the inner surface of the jaws.

145

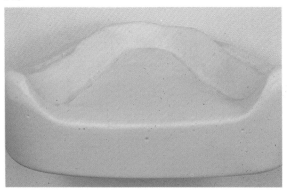

145 Model of the jaw. Impressions were obtained of the suspect's lower jaw and a model was prepared. This is viewed from the same aspect as the model in **144** and indicates that although there has been shrinkage of the jaw, the overall outline and features are similar to the model prepared from the denture.

146 Upper denture of the accused man. When he was apprehended the accused man was wearing only an upper denture. Initial examination indicated that this upper denture had been made of material similar to the lower denture found at the scene of the crime and also that the standard of workmanship was the same. It was important to be able to show that the lower denture found at the scene of the crime was actually the 'mate' of the upper denture being worn by the accused.

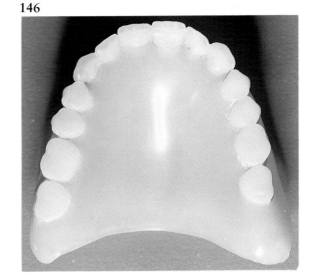

147 Matching of upper and lower dentures. Detailed examination of the upper and lower dentures showed that there were exactly corresponding facets of wear, where the upper and lower dentures had ground together during use. There can be no doubt that the lower denture found at the scene of the crime corresponded to the upper denture worn by the accused at the time of his arrest.

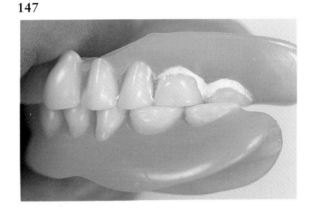

Damage to dentures and repairs

As has been shown, distinctive wear patterns may allow matching of opposed upper and lower dentures. Less frequently, distinctive wear of artificial teeth may indicate particular habits or occupations, in the same way as in natural teeth (see **46**).

Dentures made of a rigid and relatively brittle plastic can be damaged by being dropped or otherwise abused. This may result in individual teeth being dislodged, or in the denture base being broken. Repairs may then be undertaken and the presence and nature of the repairs can provide useful information for identification.

148

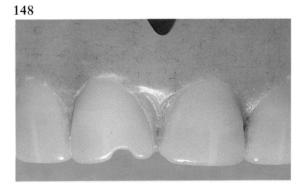

148 Notched incisor tooth. This denture from a middle-aged female shows a distinctive notch in one of the upper front teeth. Such wear is likely to be caused by something being held in the teeth or rubbing against that particular area of tooth. This could be a particular habit, or perhaps occupational damage, for example a seamstress who breaks threads with her teeth.

149

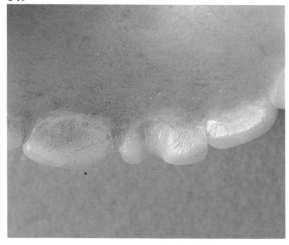

150

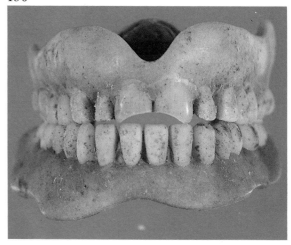

149 Distinctive tooth wear. This view is of the back surface of the tooth shown in **148**. It indicates that there is a groove on the back of the tooth in continuity with the notch in the biting edge. This suggested that the lady might have been a hairdresser who was in the habit of opening hairgrips with her teeth during her daily work.

150 Worn and repaired denture. This denture was found on the unidentified body of a man who had been burned in a fire. Dentures can survive surprisingly well in fires provided they are not directly exposed to the flames. There is wear of the upper central incisors which was later matched with a particular pipe smoked by a known missing person. The part of the acrylic baseplate related to the upper front teeth is a slightly different shade from the rest of the denture, indicating that it has been damaged and then repaired.

151

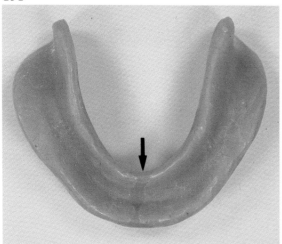

152

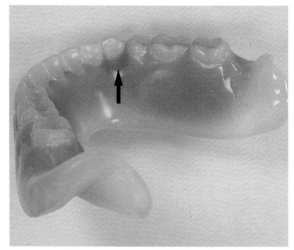

151 Repair to lower denture base. This lower denture has been broken near the midline, and repaired with acrylic. The view from the fitting surface makes the site of the repair (arrow) much more obvious than was evident on the polished surface. The original baseplate on either side of the fracture has been cut back and the repair has been effected with self-curing acrylic.

152 Extensive modification of denture. The appliance illustrated has been rebased. In this technique the original fitting surface of the denture is removed, but the tooth-bearing part is retained. New casts of the jaws are prepared and a new denture base is made which accommodates changes caused by the shrinkage of the denture-bearing parts of the jaws. At the same time a repair was done in which a tooth was reattached with self-cure acrylic (arrow).

Chapter 10
Partial dentures and orthodontic appliances

The term 'partial denture' is used when the appliance replaces missing teeth in one jaw in a patient who retains some natural teeth. Partial dentures are much more variable than full dentures both in design and in the materials used in their construction.

The possibilities for identification from partial dentures are similar to those from full dentures. However, for several reasons both ante-mortem records and the dentist's memory of individual cases are likely to be better in the case of partial dentures.

Decisions about which teeth should be replaced by the denture may mean that the dentist has to consider extraction of some teeth and preparation of other teeth or restorations adjacent to the denture. The dentist prescribes the design of the denture for the technician and specifies the materials and teeth to be used. These details are likely to be noted on the dentist's record. The nature and quality of the workmanship may also indicate the type of laboratory in which the denture was made.

Partial denture construction

The simplest types of partial denture consist of an acrylic baseplate and acrylic teeth. This may be made without any clasps on the remaining teeth, or a wide variety of metal clasps may be used to aid retention. A better alternative to a plastic partial denture base in many cases is a metal base which can be made to cover much less normal tissue. In special cases highly complex designs of dentures can be used to replace teeth in particular situations or to modify an individual mouth, for example by propping the jaws open.

153

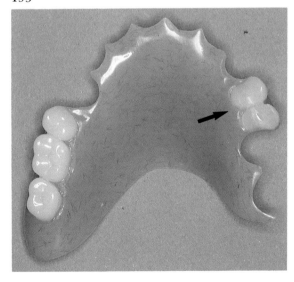

153 **Acrylic partial denture.** This is a simple partial denture replacing five upper teeth. The baseplate fits around the necks of the remaining natural teeth. A distinctive feature in this case is that two artificial teeth (arrow) have been used to fill the gap caused by one missing tooth, because the gap was greater than the size of one tooth.

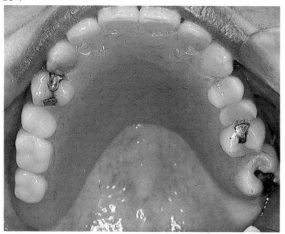

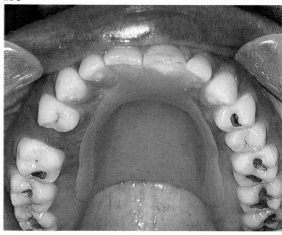

154   Acrylic partial denture. This is the denture shown in **153** in the mouth, confirming the nature of the construction. It is possible from examination of the denture alone to determine which natural teeth would have been present in the mouth. This is a poor design of denture because it causes damage to the soft tissues, particularly at the necks of the remaining teeth. It is often possible when examining a partially dentate mouth to determine whether or not a denture has been worn.

155   Spoon denture. This type of denture can be used to replace a single upper front tooth. The denture fits into the palate but does not make contact with the teeth other than those adjacent to the gap being filled. This type of denture has very limited retention in the mouth, being largely controlled by the tongue. Often the denture is even smaller than the case shown and could readily be dislodged. In a forensic case, this might require a search to be conducted in the surrounding area and in the windpipe, in case the denture had been inhaled. Some authorities recommend that such dentures should include radiopaque material to facilitate radiographic location of inhaled small plates.

156

157

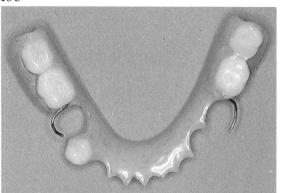

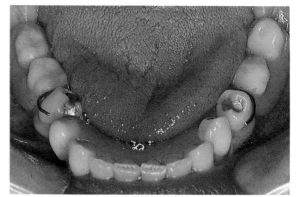

156   Acrylic denture with metal clasps. This lower denture replacing five teeth is constructed with an acrylic baseplate and acrylic teeth. In order to aid retention, two metal clasps have been incorporated. These are related to two natural teeth and they are designed so that the flexible ends of the clasps engage undercuts on the teeth.

157   Acrylic denture with metal clasps. The view in the mouth of the denture illustrated in **156** shows the metal clasps grasping the natural teeth. These are clasps of inexpensive construction in stainless steel wire. Better quality clasps may be cast in gold or non-precious metal and can be of very varied design. Although clasps are designed to be as inconspicuous as possible, they can sometimes be detected in 'toothy snapshots' and are therefore of value when such photographs are being used as part of the ante-mortem record for identification.

158 Cast metal partial denture. This partial upper denture has a cast chrome cobalt base which is tooth borne. Three artificial teeth are present, attached to the metal base by pink acrylic. The metal casting includes clasps around some teeth. Occlusal rests (arrows) are also present on some teeth to support the denture. The natural teeth involved in such cases are often specially prepared to support the occlusal rests.

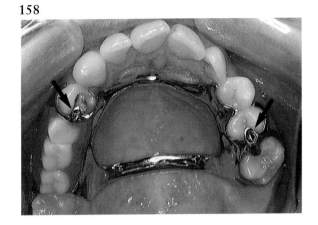

Complex partial dentures

A wide variety of complex partial denture designs is available to meet particular clinical problems. One complex case is illustrated by way of an example.

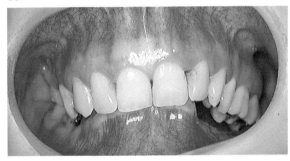

159 Patient with deep overbite. This patient has natural upper teeth and some natural lower teeth. The upper and lower front teeth overlap to a considerable extent when the patient closes her teeth together and this causes damage to the soft tissues of the gums. The clinical problem is to replace the missing lower teeth with a denture and at the same time alter the way the patient bites in order to avoid the damage to the gums.

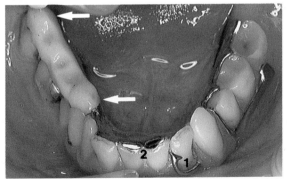

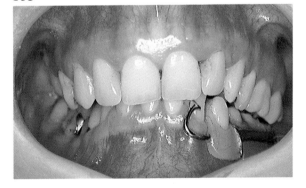

160 Complex partial denture. The denture has a cast chrome cobalt metal base that includes a clasp (1) and rests on the incisal edges of the lower central incisors (2). Artificial teeth are present on the patient's left. In order to open the bite and prevent gum damage, the occlusal surfaces of the natural teeth on the patient's right have been covered (arrows). This is known as an overdenture.

161 Correction of overbite. Comparison with 159 shows how the effect of the overdenture has been to 'prop open' the patient's jaws slightly, thus stopping the anterior teeth from damaging the gums. The cast metal clasp is clearly seen.

Identification from partial dentures

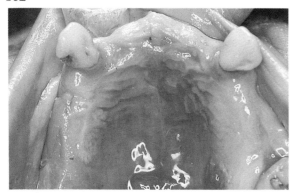

162   Partially dentate mouth. The body of a murdered woman was found in undergrowth a few days after her death. Three upper teeth were present and the condition of the soft tissues of the palate and adjacent to the teeth suggested that a denture had probably been worn. A search of the area around the body resulted in the finding of an acrylic partial upper denture.

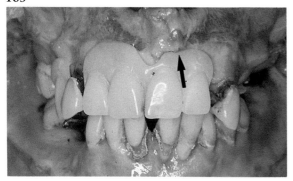

163   Fitting the denture to the body. The denture was inserted into the excised maxilla of the body to demonstrate that it bore the missing teeth and that it had been prescribed for the victim. Facets on the palatal side of the acrylic incisors matched the lower standing incisors, confirming that it had been worn by the woman. A further distinctive feature was evident where part of the flange of the denture (arrow) had been modified to avoid irritation to an unusual bony prominence.

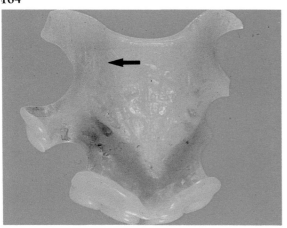

164   Features of the denture. This view of the fitting surface of the denture indicates that it had been made at a time when the patient had several more teeth than were evident in the body. Close examination revealed some indistinct marking on part of the denture (arrow).

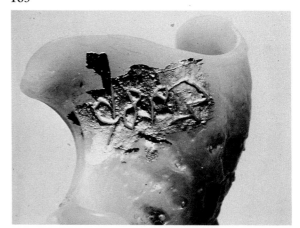

165   Marks on denture. The marks on the denture base were difficult to see. Graphite disclosing powder was applied to the area and this highlighted a prescription code which had been cut into the stone model on which the denture was processed. This was identified as a marking code used in a local long-stay hospital and from their records the name of the owner was traced.

Orthodontic treatment

Orthodontic treatment is used to correct abnormalities of the position, angulation or rotation of teeth. This is usually done in adolescence, but an increasing amount of orthodontic treatment is undertaken in young adults. Often teeth have to be extracted to allow space for the remaining teeth to be properly aligned. Sometimes the tooth movement can be achieved by removable appliances which are similar to partial dentures but which carry springs or other devices to apply pressure to individual teeth to achieve the desired movement. Alternatively, a fixed appliance can be used in which the movement is achieved by devices attached directly to the teeth.

The preparatory stages of orthodontic treatment involve careful analysis, including radiographs and study models of the teeth. Radiographs and models will also be available in most cases at the conclusion of treatment and will be retained as part of the dentist's record (see Chapter 12).

Orthodontic appliances

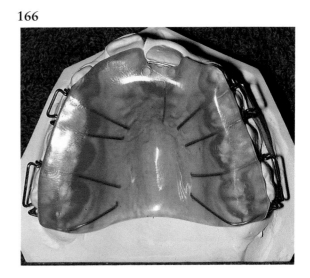

166 Removable appliance. The appliance consists of an acrylic baseplate with clasps on some teeth and an active component to move the upper left central incisor towards the lip. It is shown on a dental stone model of the teeth, which would be retained with the patient's records.

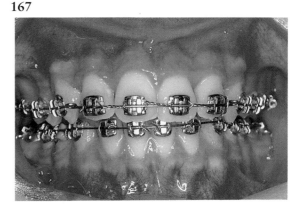

167 Fixed orthodontic appliance. In this case the appliance is fixed directly to the teeth and would be worn for many months. In the UK this type of treatment is likely to be undertaken by consultant orthodontists in hospitals or in a small number of specialist practices. Much more complex forms of treatment can be achieved with fixed appliances than with removable appliances.

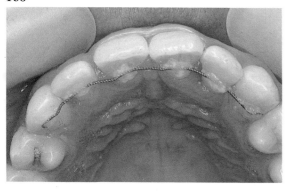

168 Orthodontic retainer. On completion of orthodontic treatment it may be necessary to ensure that the teeth remain in their new position. A retainer of the type shown may be cemented to the back surfaces of the teeth for several years in order to prevent unwanted tooth movement.

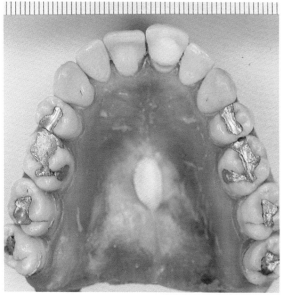

169 Recognition of previous orthodontic treatment. The upper jaw from an unidentified body shows apparently well aligned teeth in a regular arch. The upper first premolars on each side are missing. A similar situation existed in the lower jaw, and it was quite clear that the individual had previously been treated with an orthodontic fixed appliance.

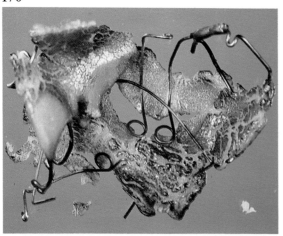

170 Recognition of burnt appliance. The tongue and lips will often protect the contents of the oral cavity if a corpse is incinerated. In this case the acrylic baseplate of an orthodontic appliance was sufficiently intact to be recognizable, which helped in identification.

Chapter 11
Laboratory procedures

Most forensic dental investigations entail the application of a sound knowledge of the general principles of dentistry and basic dental science to problems in which there is a medicolegal interest. Usually the clinical findings will provide a basis for comparison of this information with that contained in previous dental or medical records. The presence or absence of restorations and their design and type, the eruption status of the individual, the presence of pathological conditions or unusual characteristics of the jaws and teeth may usually be ascertained by straightforward but detailed examination of the tissues or by the use of suitable radiographs. There will, however, be cases presented to the forensic dentist where more sophisticated techniques are required. The teeth, the surrounding tissues, the cells associated with them and the fluids maintaining their viability can all be examined in the laboratory to yield information which cannot be obtained by gross observation. Scientific techniques should be well tried and tested and be generally acceptable to the scientific community, and in particular to the dental community. It is not usually appropriate to use new techniques, the reliability of which, in the forensic situation, may be unacceptable. Changes occurring after death, putrefaction of the tissues and the effect of the environment frequently affect the validity of laboratory techniques, and the effect of these variables should be known and appreciated by an investigator. In general, laboratory methods will supplement and support evidence acquired in a more routine manner, but the forensic dentist must be prepared to explain in detail to the courts why the investigations were necessary and to be frank and open about their limitations.

Recognition of tissues

It is an axiom of scene-of-crime activity that any evidence, however inexplicable, should be collected and carefully preserved for future study. Those responsible should not discard fragments of material because they are not familiar with their origin. Investigating officers should bear in mind that it may be possible to extract useful information from seemingly useless fragments of material and that if there is any possibility that these may have originated from the oral region then it may be worthwhile seeking the advice of a forensic dentist.

171

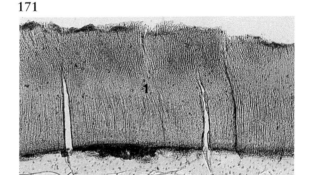

171 Light microscopy of tooth enamel. This specimen was retrieved from the boot of a car in which it was thought possible that a body had been transported following an attempt to cremate it. Although it looked like a small chip of hard stone a few millimetres in size, microscopy revealed that tooth enamel (1) was present. When teeth are cremated the dentine core of the tooth frequently expands shattering off the enamel in small pieces. Microscopic recognition of such a fragment was clearly an important piece of evidence relating fragments of a body to the vehicle in question.

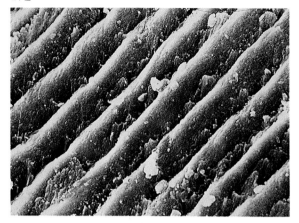

172 Scanning electron microscopy. Fragments of teeth are often extremely friable and difficult to section for light microscopy, but may sometimes be prepared in such a way that examination in the scanning electron microscope is possible. This fragment of hard material found in the depths of a human bite mark consists of typical tooth enamel prisms, indicating that suspects with intact anterior teeth could not have been involved in the biting episode. Recognition of artefacts of this nature as dental tissues is clearly essential before further progress can be made.

173

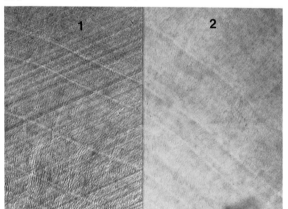

173 Incremental growth patterns. A section of human enamel (1), was discovered in the examination of a bite mark on the upper arm of a female murder victim. Some months after the tragedy the body of a male suicide victim was discovered and it was noticed that a small fragment was missing from the upper left central incisor. A section of tooth was prepared (2). The faint curved lines running diagonally are incremental growth patterns built into the enamel of this tooth during its development many years previously. They are associated with minor changes in physiological activity during the laying down of the hard tissues of the tooth and are said to be unique to each individual. These growth lines match in the tooth fragment (1) and the sectioned tooth (2), strongly suggesting that the fragment originated from this tooth.

174

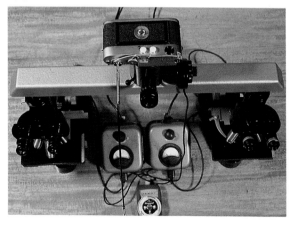

174 Comparison microscope. This is a device allowing two sections or specimens (see **173**) to be viewed simultaneously at exactly the same magnification so that a correlation can be tested between the two. The same principle is used in a comparison between rifling marks on bullets fired from the same gun. In the case of enamel specimens it is necessary to arrange that the portion of enamel studied from the fragment was developing at the same time as the portion studied from the remainder of the tooth in order that the growth lines will be coincident. The investigator should therefore be fully conversant with the developmental stages of the human dentition.

Species, sex and serology

Small fragments of bones or teeth may retain sufficient characteristics to allow determination of species of origin, sex and blood or tissue groupings to be carried out in the laboratory. Success depends on the freshness of the specimen and whether tooth fragments consist of enamel or dentine.

175 **Bone structure.** Some authorities have suggested that the structure of bone in different animals varies to such an extent that species determinations can be made on ground or demineralized sections. There are said to be distinct differences in the size and distribution of the haversian canals in the compact bone of different animal types. As a general rule, the haversian canals are said to be larger in size but fewer in number in human material compared with that of a dog or cat. This example is of the alveolar bone surrounding a human molar tooth.

175

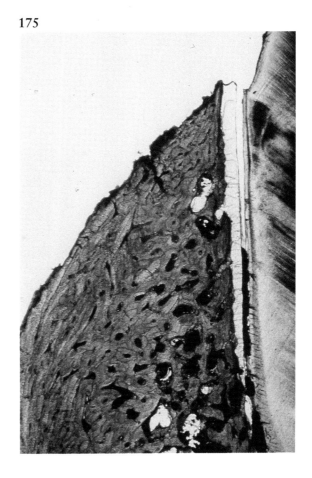

176 Morphology. This tooth fragment (1) was discovered in a cucumber sandwich. The tooth (2) is the second lower premolar of the domestic pig, highlighting the portion thought to correspond to the unknown fragment. Superimposition (3) shows the general shape and morphological characteristics such as the ridges on the lingual side of the crown are alike in both the fragment and the whole tooth.

176

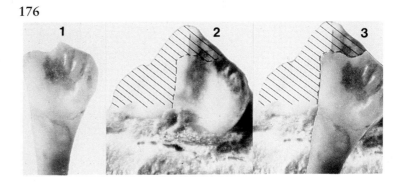

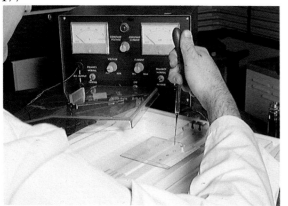

177 Serology for species identification. Although the enamel of a tooth contains very little organic or living material, the dentine from the core of the tooth may contain not only body fluids but in some circumstances processes of living cells. A fragment containing less than one cubic millimetre of dentine will contain identifiable antigens unique to a particular species. The fluid can be compared with known antibodies raised in the laboratory against a range of animals using countercurrent electrophoresis.

178

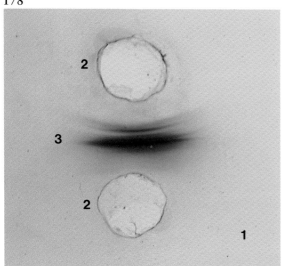

178 Precipitation reaction. Aliquots of the fluid extracted from the dentine are placed in one line of circular wells cut in the electrophoresis gel (1). Suitably diluted antibodies from various known species are placed in adjacent wells about 1 mm distant (2). A positive reaction occurs only where the correct species antibody has been chosen to test against the unknown extracted fluid, and this positive reaction results in a stainable precipitation in the gel (3). It has been shown that positive reactions may be achieved on dentinal fluids extracted from teeth up to nine months after death. The technique is demanding, as dilution factors are critical to the success of this particular test.

179

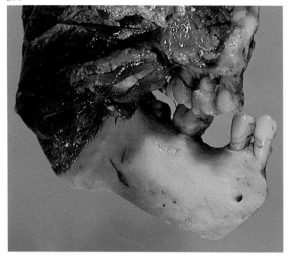

179 Sex determination from fragments. Certain parts of the body, particularly the pelvis, may have clear characteristics related to one of the sexes, and even in the skull there may be features which suggest maleness or femaleness (see **82** to **86**). Such features may be absent or indeterminate, and in these cases laboratory techniques offer a solution. This fragment of a human skull was discovered following an accident with a ship's propeller and, as has already been mentioned, the teeth may often survive. Although teeth are largely composed of hard tissues, the pulp or nerve inside the tooth and the supporting tissues around it are cellular in nature. Removal of a few of the cells from either the external surface of the tooth or preferably from inside the pulp chambers will usually provide enough tissue for a sex determination to be made.

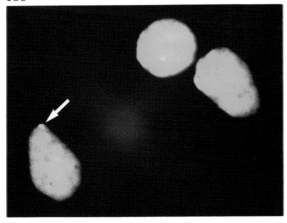

180 The Y chromosome. The cellular remnants are smeared on a microscope slide and fixed using standard cytological methods. Even months after death these cells will contain nuclear or chromatin material. In the case of the male an X and Y chromosome would be expected, whereas in the case of the female two X chromosomes are found. Certain dyes have an affinity for the Y chromosome and they may be made fluorescent, allowing demonstration under the microscope using ultraviolet light. These cells have been subjected to such a staining technique and the bright green fluorescent spot can be seen in each nucleus, indicating that Y chromosome material was present. False positives arising from debris (arrow) are a problem with this technique. Recently, more sophisticated methods of DNA analysis from human or animal cells have been developed and in the future it is to be expected that the science of molecular biology will play an increasing role in forensic investigations.

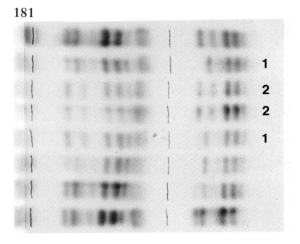

181 Analysis of body fluids. The analysis of saliva deposits left on cigarette butts, on clothing or in human bite marks is a standard forensic technique and is based on determination of the salivary enzyme amylase. A similar approach may be used to detect body fluids in tooth fragments left at the scene of a crime. Blood grouping from small fragments of teeth has been shown to be unreliable, especially when considerable time has elapsed since the event. However, phosphoglucomutase (PGM) enzymes may be extracted from small fragments of dentine up to some months after death and can be typed using electrophoresis (see 177). The proteins in the fluid are characterized by their relative mobility in electrophoretic gels and the bands of protein so produced can be stained and compared with known PGM enzyme activity. Two different types of enzymes (1 and 2) are indicated by the stained bands and a PGM grouping which is different from that of a suspect will eliminate him or her from the enquiry.

Determination of age

If a body cannot be aged from the stage of development of the teeth it may be possible to use biochemical methods.

182 Amino acids in collagen. It has recently been shown that the collagen which forms a high proportion of the dentine is constructed from amino acids which, when they are first incorporated, are of the levo or left-handed enantiomer variety. Once these amino acids have become fixed in the dentine of the tooth they undergo a slow and irreversible change to dextro or right-handed enantiomers, and the ratio between these two types is a measure of the time elapsed since the amino acids were first incorporated into the tooth. This graph shows that the age calculated from the ratio of aspartic acid types closely fits the chronological age in six bodies of known elapsed time since death. These techniques are still in the developmental stage but give an indication of the direction in which basic dental science may be able to aid the forensic dentist in the future.

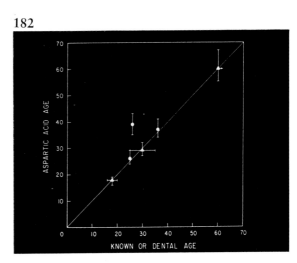

Estimation of time since death

Determination of time of death is still one of the unsolved problems in forensic pathology. The forensic dentist has nothing to offer in this respect in the immediate post-death period, but as time goes by certain changes can occur in the teeth which may help.

183

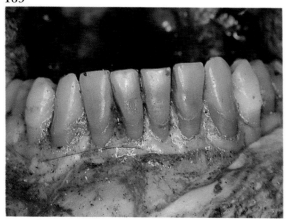

183 Pink teeth. In some bodies the teeth acquire a pink to purple discoloration which clearly represents a post-mortem change. Our knowledge of this phenomenon is still incomplete, but the evidence suggests that pink teeth are not apparent in the first one and a half to two weeks after death. It has been suggested that violent death such as strangulation may raise the venous pressure immediately before death to such an extent that small capillaries in the pulps of the teeth rupture releasing red blood cells into the pulp and possibly into the dentinal tubules. In forensic practice the phenomenon is most frequently seen in victims of drowning, in whom the head frequently lies in a dependent position. The subsequently developing pink teeth may be analogous to post-mortem lividity stains at the most dependent parts of the body.

184

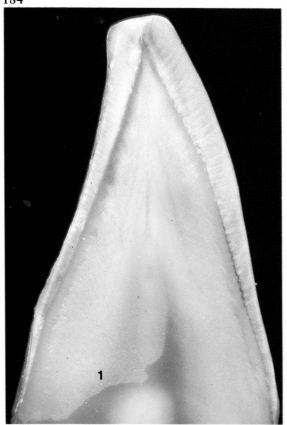

184 Microscopic section of pink tooth. The pigment is contained within the dentine (1) and is most strongly seen surrounding the pulp of the tooth. This accords with the suggestion that blood products pass into the dentinal tubules from the blood vessels. Chemical analysis of the pink material has confirmed that complex blood breakdown products are involved and these can be extracted and characterized biochemically, or they can be demonstrated in the dentinal tubules using suitable histochemical techniques. As more cases of this phenomenon are studied, the relationships between cause and time of death and the development of pink teeth may become clearer, enabling the forensic dentist to contribute in a small way to this perplexing problem.

Wound healing

In identification procedures or in investigations of sudden death or assault, an opinion is frequently sought on the time elapsed since a particular injury. The rate at which wounds heal depends upon several factors, notably the absence or presence of infection and the size of the initial wound. A histological section through the healing wound will yield much information as to the time since its infliction.

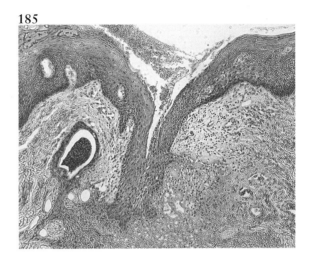

185 Epithelial wound healing. This injury was a clean incision with a knife through the lining of the mouth, and the epithelium has migrated along the depth of the wound and has achieved fusion at the base of the injury. In order for the cells to proliferate and migrate sufficiently for this to have occurred, several days must have elapsed since the incision was made. Observable inflammatory reaction to a wound may take from a few hours up to 24 hours to develop. The presence of bleeding strongly suggests that wounding occurred before death. Bruises in or around the mouth or associated with bite marks almost certainly indicate that injury preceded death, although it has been shown that marks similar to bruises can occasionally be produced by very severe trauma to tissues in the post-mortem period.

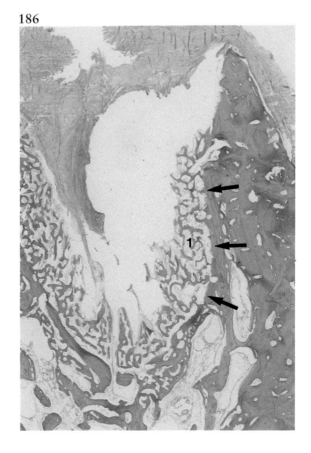

186 Healing extraction wounds. When comparisons are to be made between the status of a mouth at the time of death and previous dental records, clinical investigation of an extraction socket or its appearance on a radiograph may be misleading as to the time when the tooth was extracted. In general, the soft tissues start healing in the first few hours after extraction but epithelialization is not usually complete for two to three weeks. The outline of a bony socket may remain within the mandible or maxilla for many months or occasionally years after the tooth was removed, so that a precise dating may be impossible. A histological section will reveal the presence or absence of either woven or adult bone, thus enabling a more accurate estimate to be made of time elapsed since the surgical intervention. In the example shown the outline of the original socket (arrows) is evident, and woven bone (1) is being laid down.

Tooth characteristics

The hard tissues of the permanent teeth, particularly the enamel and dentine, are laid down between birth and the end of the second decade, depending upon which tooth is being considered. Serious disturbances caused by disease or genetic abnormalities may influence the manner in which these hard tissues are laid down, and imperfections so caused will be present in the tooth for the remainder of its existence. Such disturbances may not always be clearly visible clinically, so microscopic examination is required to reveal them.

187

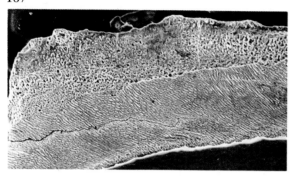

187 Enamel hypoplasia. In this scanning electron micrograph of a deciduous tooth the outer enamel is markedly disorganized as a result of hypoplasia. This condition was hereditary, but it appears to affect the enamel produced after birth more markedly than that produced before birth. Malformations such as this found either in the child or in the adult dentition are relatively rare and should be traceable to a family with a known similar incidence of this condition.

188

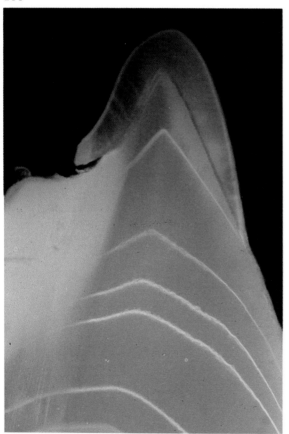

188 Drug therapy. Not only do disease processes themselves affect the development of the teeth, but so also may the use of certain drugs in the treatment of these conditions. Tetracycline antibiotics cause discoloration of the developing teeth by binding to the hydroxyapatite crystals being laid down in the forming dentine or enamel. These drugs are fluorescent in ultraviolet light and are visible on ground sections through the tooth. In some children multiple doses have been used, and in this case the results of at least five independent courses of treatment can be seen as fluorescent lines in the dentine. When suitable allowance is made for the rate of enamel and dentine formation, the period of time elapsed between the individual courses of treatment can be estimated, enabling a comparison to be made with previous medical records.

189 Dental instrumentation. Not all defects in the dental hard tissues are caused by natural disease. The structure of a tooth may be radically changed by the application of various dental instruments used in the preparation of teeth to accept fillings or restorations of various types. The dentine of this tooth has been cut away using a rotary instrument in order to prepare it for the attachment of a post crown. The marks are typical of those produced by a fast rotating diamond stone and differ from those produced by other rotating instruments. As dental surgeons often have a predilection for a particular type of instrument, evidence of this nature may be useful if the dentist can be traced.

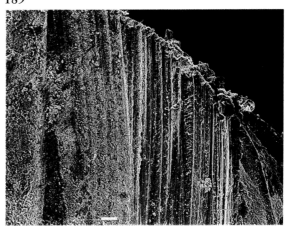

Bite mark analysis

On occasions, bite marks found on a murder or assault victim are insufficiently defined for it to be certain that a human bite has occurred. Bleeding into the tissues would be expected resulting in a bruise, both at the point of application of the individual teeth and subsequent to pressure from the lips and tongue. There may also be disruption of the underlying fibres of the connective tissue. In addition, in a severe bite the overlying epithelium may have been penetrated. Where the victim died following the biting, the method of storage of the body may markedly influence the demonstration of some of these features histologically.

190 Histology of a bite mark. This section of skin and underlying connective tissue is taken from the nipple of a murdered rape victim. The section reveals loss of the overlying epithelium from the abrasive activity of the incisor teeth of the assailant and large oedematous spaces in the underlying connective tissue. In routinely stained sections no evidence of bruising was visible, so that the firm diagnosis of a bite was thrown into considerable doubt. The body had been preserved by freezing at −16°C and had subsequently been thawed before being examined. Freezing lyses red blood cells, and in this section a special technique has been used resulting in a positive blue stain for haem breakdown products. The major features of a human bite were therefore present and the investigation proceeded with that knowledge.

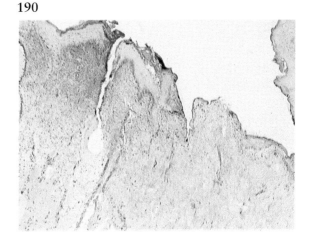

190

Chapter 12
Ante-mortem records and comparisons

With the possible exception of the few cases where a denture with a name is found, it is highly unlikely that an unknown body would be identified by dental means simply from examination of the corpse. In every other case the post-mortem findings have to be compared with some existing data on the individual thought to be involved in order to establish an identification.

The obvious records to use for dental identification are those of dentists who have treated or examined the individual during life. The dental expert needs to be aware of a number of factors in relation to such records before using them for comparison with post-mortem records.

The first problem may be in obtaining dental records. In the UK most dental treatment is done under the National Health Service. For this service the dentist is required to do a basic charting of the patient's mouth, recording the teeth missing and the teeth replaced by a denture. There is no statutory requirement to chart the existing restorations. When the dentist has completed a course of treatment, a duplicate record is submitted, with a list of the treatment which has been undertaken, to the national Dental Estimates Board for payment. Some items require prior approval, for which the dentist submits details before undertaking the treatment. Records are therefore held by both the dentist and the Dental Estimates Board. The dentist is required to retain a copy of the record for only two to five years, depending on the nature of the treatment given. The Dental Estimates board retain their copies of the records for only a few years.

Fortunately, many dentists, whether in NHS or private practice, retain much fuller records for longer than the required minimum, and this is obviously helpful in forensic dental terms. Certain types of people are likely to have more detailed records which are retained for a long time, for example those in the Armed Services, and those in certain 'high risk' categories, such as some airline personnel, are subject to regular dental examinations and good records of these are retained.

The starting point in the search for ante-mortem dental records is the name of the individual who might be involved. Records can then be sought from appropriate sources. It is worth remembering that the individual patient may attend several dentists over a lifetime, and only by obtaining records from each of these can a full record of the mouth be compiled.

In cases where identity has not been established, dental records of a body are sometimes circulated in dental professional journals in the hope of finding a dentist who might recognize the mouth of the deceased. This is rarely successful, but the chances of success can be improved by ensuring that the optimum records are circulated.

If the dental records are obtained it is important that the ante-mortem and post-mortem records are compared by a dentist. Dental records often contain errors which might appear to someone not fully conversant with such records to preclude a positive identification.

In the absence of adequate formal dental records, there are other sources of ante-mortem dental details which can either supplement or replace them. These include radiographs in medical records, 'toothy' photographs, or dental details recalled by people who knew the individual thought to be the unidentified body.

Dental charting

RIGHT								LEFT							
8	7	6	5	4	3	2	1	1	2	3	4	5	6	7	8
8	7	6	5	4	3	2	1	1	2	3	4	5	6	7	8

191 Dental Estimates Board record. The basic charting required of NHS dentists in the UK is to indicate which teeth are missing by scoring through the appropriate tooth on the chart. The dentist is also required to indicate which teeth are replaced by a denture. There is no statutory requirement to chart which fillings are already present when the patient presents for a course of treatment. Note that the chart divides the mouth into four quadrants each with eight teeth. The convention is that the teeth are charted as seen by the dentist looking at the patient from the front. The teeth on the patient's right side therefore appear on the left hand side of the chart. Individual teeth may be designated by the quadrant symbol and number: 1⏌, for example, is the upper right central incisor. Deciduous or baby teeth are charted using the letters A to E in each quadrant instead of numbers.

192

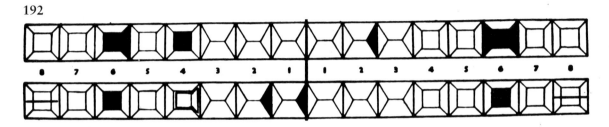

192 Dental chart. The record most frequently used by dentists for their own practice purposes contains diagrammatic representations of the teeth. A surface blocked out on the record indicates that there is a filling involving that surface. The upper left first molar has an MOD filling (see **52**). A cavity is marked by highlighting the surface but not blocking it out. The lower right first premolar has an MO cavity. A line through the diagram indicates a missing tooth. The disadvantage of such records is that they are diagrammatic and give no information as to the size and shape of fillings. An alternative form of dental record using anatomically correct tooth shapes (see **13**) rather than diagrams is favoured in some countries.

193

RIGHT								LEFT							
18	17	16	15	14	13	12	11	21	22	23	24	25	26	27	28
48	47	46	45	44	43	42	41	31	32	33	34	35	36	37	38

193 Other charting systems. Although the anatomical description of teeth is essentially the same in different countries, the systems of designation used in dental records show considerable variation. This can pose particular problems in mass disasters where dental records are obtained from different countries. The Federation Dentaire Internationale (FDI) has advocated the adoption of the two digit system. The quadrants are numbered 1 to 4 and the teeth 1 to 8 in each quadrant. The upper left central incisor is thus designated 21 (expressed as two one, not twenty-one). For deciduous teeth the quadrants are numbered 5 to 8 and the teeth 1 to 5 in each quadrant.

Records for an unidentified body

When the post-mortem dental examination has been completed the most difficult problem in progressing to an identification is obtaining adequate ante-mortem records. If there is no initial indication who the individual might be, a search through police records of known missing persons can be a good starting point.

194

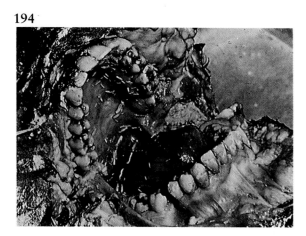

194 Unidentified body. These are the jaws, shown here partially dissected, of a middle-aged female who had committed suicide. A post-mortem charting was made. Search through police records of missing persons produced the name of a woman who might have been the unidentified body. Contact with the family provided the name of the dentist who had treated the woman, and his records were obtained.

195

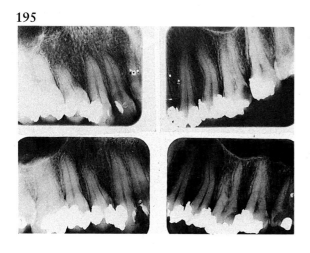

195 The dentist's record. The record for this case included radiographs. The uppermost two radiographs in the illustration are from the dentist. It was a straightforward matter to place the jaw which had been removed from the body, in the same angulation relative to the x-ray tube and produce corresponding radiographs to the dentist's views. The lower two radiographs from the body show so many points of similarity to the dentist's radiographs that there can be no doubt as to the identity of the woman. Ante-mortem radiographs are a particularly valuable component of dental records.

Variability and errors in records

Dental records from different sources can vary considerably. The case demonstrated in the following three illustrations (shown opposite) was part of a student research project into dental identification. Known deceased patients were examined at post-mortem and their mouths were charted. Then an attempt was made to see if the bodies could have been identified by dental means. Ante-mortem records were obtained from the Dental Estimates Board and from the dentist who had treated the patient. The next three illustrations show the different records of one individual.

196

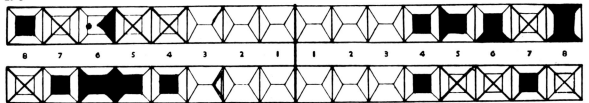

196 The students' charting. This charting undertaken by the students in the mortuary recorded four teeth missing in the upper jaw and four missing in the lower jaw. These have a cross through the relevant box on the chart. Six upper teeth and six lower teeth had restorations.

197

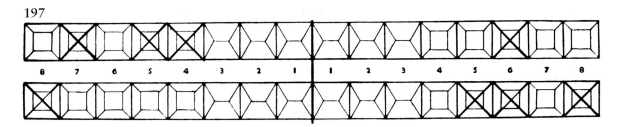

197 The Dental Estimates Board charting. The record from the Estimates Board merely noted which teeth were missing. None of these missing teeth was replaced by a denture. The charting illustrated has been prepared from the information on the Dental Estimates Board record. This record shows four upper teeth and four lower teeth missing. However, in the upper jaw, the tooth recorded as missing on the left side is the first molar, whereas the students recorded the missing tooth as the second molar. Mis-identification of molar teeth is quite often seen in records because these teeth can resemble each other closely. When molar teeth are extracted in early adolescence, the tooth developing later can grow into the space left by the extraction.

198

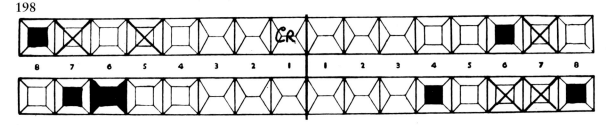

198 The dentist's record. This charting was compiled from the records of the dentist whom the patient had attended for some years. The chart shows three missing upper teeth and two missing lower teeth. Three upper teeth and four lower teeth have had restorations noted. The artificial crown on the upper right central incisor in the dentist's record was not noted by the students. This might have resulted from the difficulty of conducting a good dental examination in the mortuary as opposed to having the jaws removed and available for study in the laboratory. The other items of treatment noted in the dentist's record probably all relate to work which he had done personally. Any treatment done before the patient's first attendance, or possibly afterwards by another dentist, would not be recorded. These facts, in combination with the problems of tooth identification noted in **197**, can explain most of the apparent discrepancies between the three records in this individual.

The case illustrated in **196**, **197** and **198** highlights some of the problems of comparing dental records. It cannot be emphasized too strongly that comparisons of ante-mortem and post-mortem dental records must be done by a dental expert who is fully conversant with the limitations and potential errors in records.

Records from several dentists

A request was received in Glasgow Dental Hospital for assistance with identification of an individual thought to be one of the victims of an aircraft crash abroad. A record was held in the Dental Hospital. Records were obtained from the dentist who had referred the patient to the Dental Hospital. Subsequently the patient had attended another dentist. The next four illustrations show a part of the mouth of the patient highlighting the alterations that occurred over a period of some 14 months. They emphasize the need to obtain all recent records in order to prepare a full ante-mortem charting.

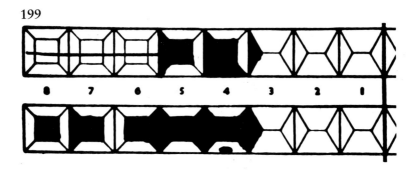

199 First dentist's record to June 1985. The patient had attended the same dentist for many years. No up-to-date charting was held by the dentist. It was possible to reconstruct a charting from the manuscript list of treatment given and a small number of radiographs. The illustration shows the part of the charting related to the posterior teeth on the right side. The upper canine and two premolar teeth have amalgam fillings. The upper molar teeth are recorded as not present. In the lower jaw all teeth from the canine posteriorly are present, each with amalgam restorations of varying sizes.

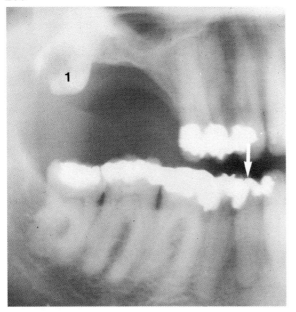

200 Dental Hospital record in June 1985. The patient had been referred for consultation to the Dental Hospital. No charting was available, but an orthopantomogram had been taken. The part of this radiograph corresponding to the charting in **199** is shown. The upper right third molar (1) was present. This tooth was unerupted, which explains why it was not noted on the dentist's record and it has been partially resorbed. In the lower jaw the first premolar (arrow) has a large restoration and there is evidence of an area of infection at the root apex. The molar teeth have large metal fillings, particularly the first molar, which appears to have an MOD amalgam as opposed to the MO amalgam noted in the dentist's record.

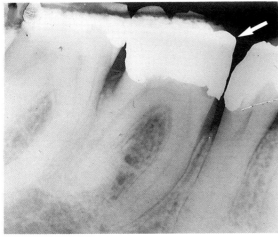

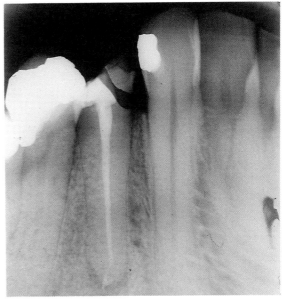

201 Second dentist's record (April 1986). The patient changed dentist and in April attended with a complaint related to the lower right first molar. The dentist removed the old amalgam filling and fitted a bonded porcelain and metal shell crown. If the contour of this restoration in the radiograph (arrow) is contrasted with the previous radiograph of the same tooth in 200, it is clear that there has been a small but significant alteration in the shape of the restoration.

202 Second dentist's records (August 1986). The lower right first premolar tooth, which had previously been noted as having an abnormality at the root apex, was root treated to remove the pulp which was the source of infection. This radiograph was taken by the dentist to confirm that the root treatment appeared satisfactory. Shortly thereafter, a crown was fitted to the tooth.

Use of multiple sources of ante-mortem dental details

In the case shown in 203 to 207, identification of a murder victim was complicated by an error in the dentist's records, and other sources of dental data were required.

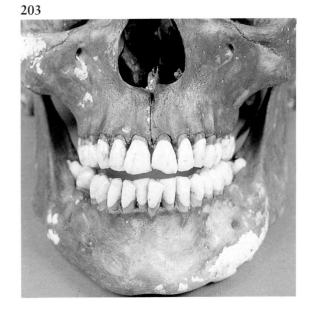

203 Unidentified body. The skeletonized body of a female was found in circumstances that suggested she had been murdered. She clearly had a good set of teeth. One upper central incisor has been damaged and there was some crowding of the lower front teeth.

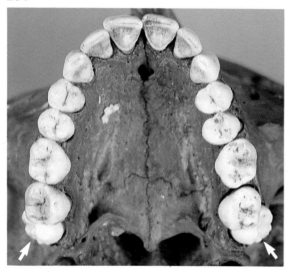

204 Upper teeth. This is an occlusal view of the upper teeth. All 16 teeth are present, although the third molar teeth (arrows) would not have been visible in the mouth during life as they were unerupted. Radiographs of these teeth showed that root formation was not quite complete, and this meant that the age could be estimated as between 21 and 23 years. There was no evidence of any dental treatment.

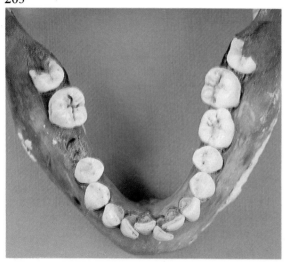

205 Lower teeth. The occlusal view of the lower teeth shows a missing lower right first molar, the socket of which is not fully healed. The dentist's record indicated that the lower right second molar tooth had been extracted a few weeks before the woman had disappeared. The two lower third molar teeth, like the upper third molars, were present but unerupted. The lower front teeth were twisted and overcrowded. The records of the individual thought to be the murdered woman showed that no fillings were present. Gum disease related to the lower front teeth had caused problems requiring treatment.

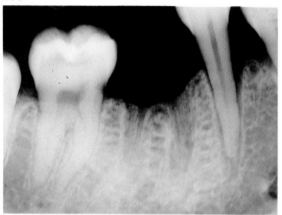

206 Radiograph of tooth socket. The radiograph of the jaws shows a partially healed socket. It is notoriously difficult to assess the time of extraction from examination of healing sockets (see **91**) but this is consistent with the socket of a tooth extracted about one to four months before death. When the original dentist examined the jaws he felt that they could have been those of his patient and that there might have been an error in the record of which tooth had been extracted. Clearly, further sources of ante-mortem dental details were required.

207 Records of the missing woman. The family were able to provide a photograph of the missing woman which showed four upper front teeth. Although the photographic quality was poor, it was evident that there was a degree of correspondence with the teeth in the body. The detail of the fractured tooth is not clear, but the family indicated that the woman was self-conscious about the damaged tooth and would mask the damage with chewing gum when being photographed. The woman's mother gave a clear history of the very twisted lower front teeth and the gum problems related to them. The additional dental evidence provided by the photograph and the mother's recollection supported the identification, although there was insufficient detail to establish identity by dental means alone. The combination of dental techniques and distinctive medical evidence allowed a positive identification to be made.

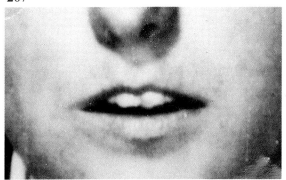

Other sources of ante-mortem records

Often, there will be difficulty in finding dental records, and then other possible sources of dental details need to be considered.

208 Hospital medical records. Some people will have general hospital records which show dental details. The radiograph illustrated was taken as part of the investigation of a fracture of the lower jaw (arrow). This view also shows considerable detail of the teeth. This type of radiographic view is likely to be held in the records of many patients who have suffered road traffic accidents or other trauma to the head and jaws. While the tooth detail shown may not always be optimal on its own for dental identification, it may be supportive, or alternatively it may be sufficient to exclude a particular identification.

208

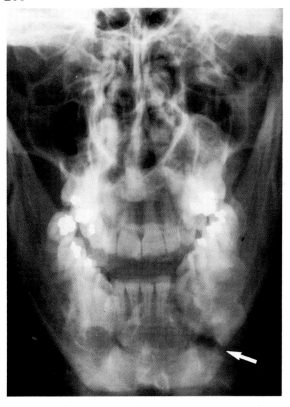

Facial comparisons and reconstruction

Attempts have been made to compare ante-mortem facial appearance with the shape of the underlying bones of the skull.

209

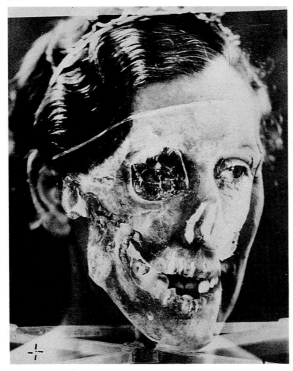

209 The Ruxton murder case. This famous 1930s case was an early example of how comparison of facial appearance to skull shape has been used to help in identification. This was done by superimposition of a facial photograph over a skull photograph printed to exactly the same size and orientation. The method enabled the skulls of two different women to be distinguished, though the technique was not actually demonstrated in the court.

210

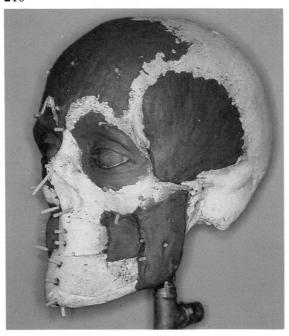

210 Facial reconstruction. It has been demonstrated that the thickness of soft tissue overlying the bones of the skull does not vary greatly between individuals. A plaster model is made of a skull requiring identification and wooden pegs are inserted at predetermined points, each one being the correct length to simulate soft tissue thickness at that point.

211 Addition of facial muscles. The contour and thickness of the muscles of facial expression are added in modelling clay, care being taken not to exceed the thickness designated by the wooden pegs at any site. The spaces between the muscles are filled in with clay to represent connective tissue, and finally the skin contour is added. In this case a deviated nasal septum and evidence of fracture of the nasal bones suggested that the nose should deviate to the right.

211

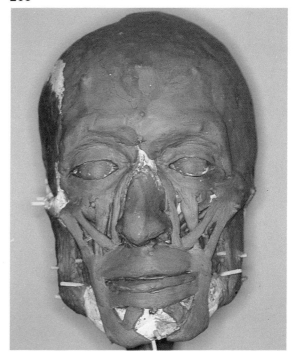

212

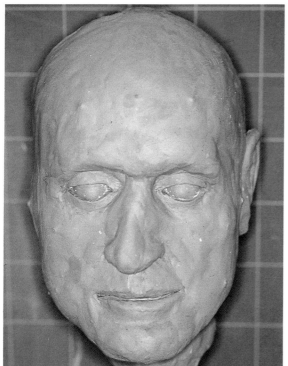

213

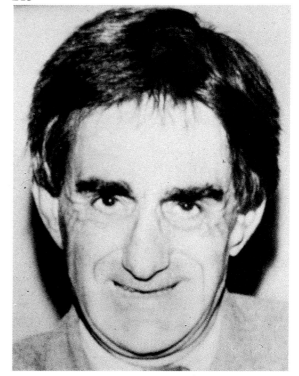

212 and 213 Skin contours. The overlying facial skin is moulded in clay so that the wooden pegs are just visible at the skin surface (212). Facial outline, contour of cheek bones and forehead are all reproduced with reasonable accuracy, although it is not possible to replace hair contour or colour. The photograph (213) is of the missing person whose skull this was believed to be and the reconstruction was made without the artist seeing this picture. There is a resemblance, though the accuracy of the method is yet to be proven.

Chapter 13
The mass disaster

Disasters involving the injury or death of a large number of people are, by their very nature, unpredictable and extremely varied in character. They may be caused by natural events, such as severe flooding, earthquake or volcanic eruption, or they may be associated with human activity, such as mass transport by rail, sea or air. Whatever the cause, mass disasters have certain features in common and these will include the destruction of property, infliction of severe injuries and multiple fatalities. A workable definition of a mass disaster is one in which the normally available forensic services would be stretched beyond acceptable limits and organized teamwork becomes a necessity.

In the event of fragmentation of bodies, specialized techniques may be required, but in general the dental techniques applied are no different to those used to deal with single bodies. The overriding problem in mass disasters is the organization of a team of specialists to deal with the particular tragedy. Although a mass disaster cannot be predicted, it is important that in geographically defined areas detailed plans are prepared, ready for execution should such a tragedy occur. Pre-planning is difficult but should aim at dealing with as many contingencies as possible, and should not only exist on paper, but should involve the training of sufficient personnel as may be reasonably appropriate. An example of such a team in the UK is that contracted to the British Airlines and responsible to the Department of Trade Accident Investigation Branch. This team is headed by a coordinator who controls pathologists, embalmers, document experts, specialists in jewellery and forensic dentists. Other countries have developed similar groups of individuals who are available at short notice and can respond promptly if needed.

In almost every situation it is advantageous to have two teams under the control of the manager, the 'site' team being involved in the collection of post-mortem information, whilst the 'home' team is responsible for the collection of ante-mortem records. In a well-planned operation there will be written procedures for each person in the team, thus preventing unnecessary duplication of effort and, more importantly, concentrating maximum expertise at the time and place where it is most needed. There have been many reports in which a high proportion of positive identifications have been achieved from the dental evidence alone or in consort with other information, but it is essential that each member recognizes the contribution of his or her colleagues to the overall success of the operation.

It is important that relatives are given the full facts of the situation as quickly as possible so that they can begin to come to terms with their loss and can take possession of the remains of their loved ones. Any procedures which remove the need for attempted visual recognition will reduce the distress and shock inevitably associated with disasters of this nature.

In this review it is possible to cover only the principles of mass disaster identification, and all the techniques of forensic dental procedure outlined in other sections of this Atlas may have to be applied in particular circumstances. The information acquired by the ante- and post-mortem teams must be regarded as entirely confidential and it should always be left solely to properly appointed people to divulge information either to the relatives or to the news media. Under no circumstances should the forensic dentists themselves communicate with anyone other than the colleagues with whom they are directly working.

Equipping the team

Because of the need for a prompt response the team should be well prepared in advance. A set of equipment should be available which is sufficiently comprehensive to deal with most major disasters.

214

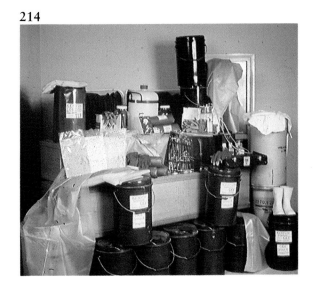

214 Dental kit. As far as the forensic dentist is concerned, the equipment previously described in **2** to **6** will be sufficient in terms of content, but it will need to be duplicated so that each active member of the dental team has his or her own supply of instruments, materials and stationery. Because large amounts of data are needed for rapid comparison, special forms are available for this purpose and must be included at the outset. In a large disaster two teams of five dentists can reasonably deal with around 150 victims in a period of five or six days, and enough equipment should be available for each group to work unhindered.

The disaster site

In a major disaster the teams responsible for the saving of human life take precedence over all other considerations. The emergency, fire, medical and ambulance services will have completed their duties before the forensic team begins its investigation.

215

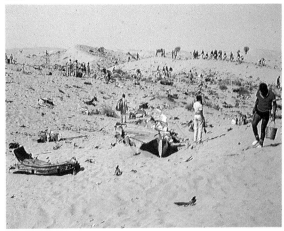

215 An air disaster. The site will have been declared safe by the appropriate authorities and it will have been cordoned off so that the whole area is enclosed and members of the public are kept far enough away to avoid them impeding the work of the team. Where forensic fragments may be difficult to locate or are spread over a wide area, such as in an air disaster, an overlapping ground search should be carried out so that as little material as possible is overlooked.

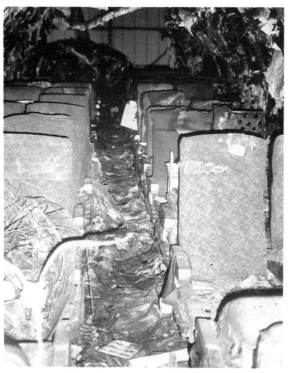

216 Location of human remains. In an enclosed area such as the cabin of an airliner or the rooms of a building a similar procedure should be followed so that the exact relationship of human remains to the surrounding furnishings or structures can be recorded both diagrammatically and photographically. One of the purposes of a comprehensive forensic investigation is to help to determine the cause of the accident and it may be important to know the position of people with particular injuries so that the sequence of events can be reconstructed.

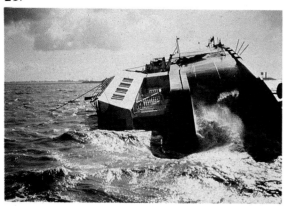

217 Disasters at sea. Some disasters may occur in places which are difficult to reach and teams of trained recovery workers will be required before identification can proceed. Where death has been caused by drowning, in the absence of forceful injury, human remains may be reasonably well preserved, particularly if ambient temperatures are low and recovery is not delayed too long. Although passenger lists may be available in some disasters involving public transport it is still important that each individual is identified. In most countries death cannot be assumed until identification is made, so disposal of a body or disposal of an estate may be delayed.

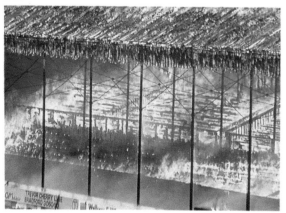

218 Major fire disasters. High intensity fires of long duration present special problems both of recognition of severely burnt bodies at the scene of the disaster and subsequent examination in the mortuary. Absolute priority is given to the saving of human life, and this is the primary role of the emergency services. Only later is consideration given to the forensic investigation of the tragedy.

219 Searching for body fragments. As each item of clothing, personal effects or body fragment is located, the position should be recorded by driving in a pre-numbered stake and any human remains should be labelled using the same code so that no doubt arises in the future as to the origin and relationship of each item. This is especially necessary if a number of badly burned bodies are located on one particular site. Searches of this nature are best carried out by trained personnel, but it may be advantageous to have the forensic dentist on hand so that if doubt arises as to the nature or importance of a particular specimen advice can be given on site.

219
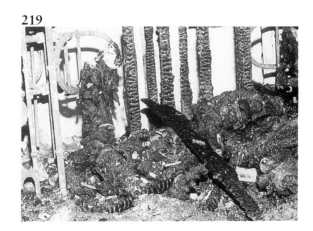

The temporary mortuary

Once the remains have been located and suitably numbered they can be removed from the site in body bags and transported for proper storage until examination can begin. In most cases the bodies will already have been moved by the time the forensic dentist and other members of the team arrive, but good facilities and arrangements at this point will greatly help the investigation team.

220 Storage of human remains. In most communities the facilities available for preservation of human bodies are limited, and few mortuaries can cope with a major disaster in addition to their normal workload. This problem is probably best solved by the provision of refrigerated trailer trucks, each of which can store about 100 bodies. The choice of site of a temporary mortuary will very much depend upon local availability. Considerable floor space is required to enable a number of tasks to continue simultaneously, and there should be separate areas where the remains can be prepared for examination, post-mortem embalming can take place and where coffins may be laid.

220
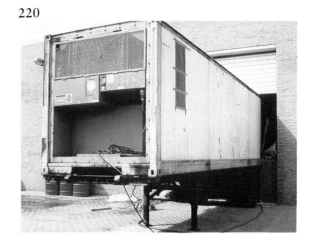

221 Post-mortem facilities. A local school, church, disused factory or public building may meet most of these requirements, but the team must be prepared to work in conditions which are less than ideal. At first sight it would seem that a local hospital would meet most of the requirements of a large scale forensic investigation, as mortuary and x-ray facilities would already be available. However, the hospital must continue its normal work and the forensic activities would need to be completely separated from the normal functions of the hospital. This can be done using tented accommodation in the grounds, but the proximity of these arrangements to the public and to busy clinical departments probably creates difficulties which outweigh the advantages.

221
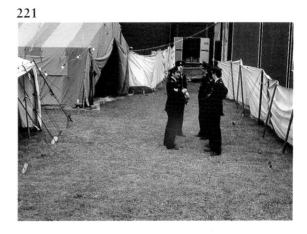

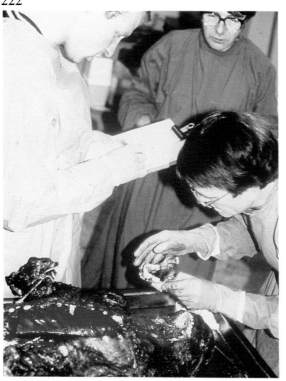

222 Planning the procedures. In the first few hours following notification of a large disaster, the team coordinator will need to make decisions concerning the number of personnel required in each section to deal with the number of bodies that are expected to be recovered. It has been estimated that two dentists working together will need about one and a half hours to complete an oral examination. The dental team leader will need to contact his or her assistants and arrange for their attendance, along with one or two additional personnel who have some experience in dental charting and, if possible, in dental radiography. Once suitable premises have been allocated and equipped for the post-mortem examinations the dental team leader's first responsibilities will be to liaise with the coordinating manager at the site. There must be a smooth flow of work from one group of experts to the next, and if more than one dental team is working the dental team leader will be responsible for coordinating their activities and making sure that all the dental findings are agreed by him or her and communicated to the project manager. Records should be kept of all procedures, including a daily log of hours worked by the teams.

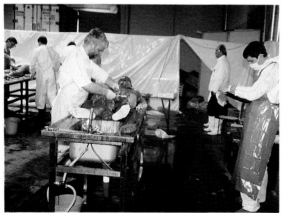

223 The post-mortem. The procedure to be followed as each cadaver is examined will depend upon the forensic pathologist's requirements. In most cases the major part of the medical examination will be completed before the remains are handed on to the dental team, but if manpower is at a premium it may be decided that some bodies will have the oral autopsy completed first. In many cases it will be necessary to remove the mandible and maxilla for closer examination (see **19** to **25**) and in general this is best left until injuries to the head and neck region have been fully examined by the medical team. As far as possible each specimen should be charted in full at the time of initial examination, as it may at best be inconvenient and at worst impossible to go back and re-examine some of the material later. Accuracy of observation and recording is paramount, which is why it is essential for two trained examiners to work in conjunction and be in complete agreement before the remains are handed on to the next team in the sequence. The mouth should be radiographed, using a portable machine, and this is most important in badly mutilated or unusual cases.

224 Impaction of facial fragments. One of the main problems of a major mass disaster is often the severe mutilation or burning of the victims. This may result in severe impaction of the dental apparatus into the soft tissues of the neck or upper thorax and observation of the oral cavity may be extremely difficult. The upper and lower jaws should be dissected out. This procedure should be carried out by a forensic dentist experienced in facial dissection so that no important features are missed. In some cases fragments of the jaws may not have been recovered at the scene of the disaster, but this should not be assumed until a careful search has been made, if necessary for each individual tooth. As the fragments are dissected free, a report to the examining pathologist should be made on any facial injuries. The pattern of these injuries may be important in determining the direction and speed of impact in the case of an air disaster or other high speed accident.

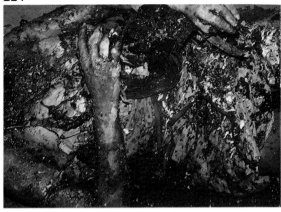

225 Embalming the remains. When the medical and dental autopsies have been completed, the human remains will have to be preserved and embalmed, and preparation made for return or repatriation of the identified remains to the next-of-kin. One of the major advantages of competent dental examination is that positive identification may be made from this alone, in conjunction with ante-mortem written records. There is therefore no need for relatives to be asked to make a visual identification from a number of mutilated and badly disfigured corpses, a situation which is known to be highly unreliable.

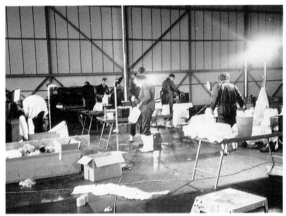

226 Repatriation of the dead. In the UK a forensic team is contracted to all of the major British airlines and their responsibility is to identify and arrange for repatriation of the dead resulting from an air disaster. The team is responsible to the Trade Accident Investigation Branch and is organized by a firm of undertakers with many years of experience in dealing with these events. The company concerned has its own team of embalmers, and following the investigations of the forensic pathologists, dental forensic experts and specialists in jewellery and documents, the human remains are placed in caskets at the scene of the investigation. The sensitive and professional manner in which these arrangements are made constitute probably the most important factor in the sad events following disasters of this magnitude. Little can ease the shock and despair suffered by those who have lost loved ones, but poor organization and insensitive handling can greatly increase the burden on those who grieve and the forensic team carries a great responsibility in expediting their task.

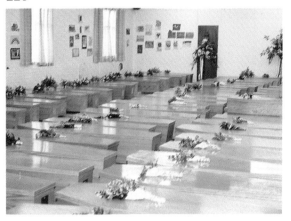

Ante-mortem records

Whilst the 'away' team is dealing with matters close to the scene of the accident, the 'home' team will be dealing with the collection of ante-mortem records. This procedure should be started as soon as possible, and from the dental point of view should be under the control of the senior dental forensic officer, who will have instructed his assistants to begin this part of the investigation before leaving for the scene.

227

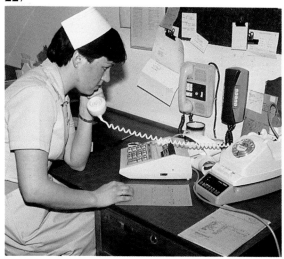

227 Liaison with the police. The ante-mortem team will work closely with the local police who have the necessary resources to sift through the enormous amount of data. They will search for written dental records, radiographs, clinical photographs and study models. The dental information will then be recorded in a form suitable for transmission to the scene of the disaster and should follow the exact procedure used by the post-mortem team. Dental records received directly from dental practitioners are rarely in a suitable form for direct comparison with the post-mortem data, so it is important that the home and away teams are entirely familiar with their techniques of recording. Two dentists should be involved in transcribing the ante-mortem data so that errors may be corrected as they arise.

228

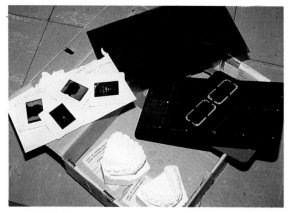

228 Transmission of data. Every available source of information should be sought, but the most useful item will be ante-mortem radiographs of the deceased. If no dental records are available, relatives or friends will have to be approached to provide descriptive information and if possible photographs, especially those showing unusual dental features. Once the data have been collected they will need to be transmitted to the post-mortem disaster team. Preliminary information may be transmitted using telex codes, a number of which have been described in the literature. More detailed ante-mortem data may be transported when convenient.

Comparison of ante- and post-mortem data

Ante-mortem information received at the disaster site may be in the form of full dental records, preliminary telexed information or in some cases computer data. The final task of the site team is to compare the ante-mortem data with the post-mortem data acquired from examination of the human remains.

229

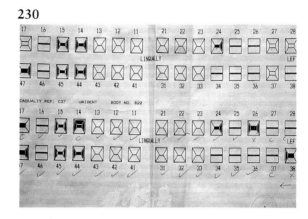

229 Preliminary comparison. The task is simplified if the data from ante-mortem records for each individual are recorded on a single form that is exactly the same as the form used by the post-mortem team. A useful preliminary approach is then to record on a large master plan unusual dental features which are unlikely to be present in more than one individual. In the case illustrated here, crowns and bridges alone have been recorded. If the information is computerized, suitable programming will allow the operator to compare large amounts of data very rapidly, but it is difficult to make allowances for errors in recording. The experience of many teams has been that manual sorting may be more reliable at present. It is still the responsibility of the forensic dentists at the scene to sift through all positive comparisons, and final identification should always be made by the expert.

231 The final report. Some authorities have suggested that ante-mortem information should be recorded on a transparent sheet in one colour, while post-mortem dental details are recorded on a similar transparent sheet using a different colour. The two sheets can then be superimposed for comparison. It has been suggested that there should be 12 concordant features before a positive identification is made, but in the final event the experience of the dental investigators will be found most important and the decision of a positive identification must finally be theirs. The final report should include details of the post-mortem and ante-mortem dental records, and to these should be added the comparison sheet on which the identification is made. In those cases where positive identification has proved impossible the only recourse is to identify by exclusion. This can be done only where the names of all the individuals concerned in a disaster are known at the outset and where the correct number of bodies has been found.

230

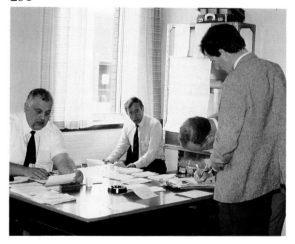

230 Detailed comparison. Once initial comparisons have been made the detailed dental records prepared by the ante- and post-mortem teams should be compared directly. The ante-mortem record is placed above the post-mortem record and it can be seen that there are discrepancies in this particular case. These discrepancies have a satisfactory professional explanation, as fillings may have been placed since the ante-mortem records were made. Where there are discrepancies which cannot be satisfactorily explained, for example where a number of teeth are present in the body but have been recorded as extracted in the ante-mortem records, a zero should be used to indicate an eliminating comparison. Where the records agree entirely a figure one should be recorded. Simple classifications of this kind will aid the comparison procedure.

231

Chapter 14
Bite marks in flesh

The term 'bite mark' is used rather loosely to describe a mark caused by the teeth alone, or the teeth in combination with other mouth parts. Bite marks can be found in flesh, foodstuffs and less frequently in a variety of other materials.

The bite marks in flesh with which the forensic dentist is likely to be concerned are most frequently found on the body of the victim. However, attack victims may attempt to defend themselves by biting their assailant. A bite mark may also be self-inflicted, either deliberately or involuntarily, for example by a hand being pressed against the victim's mouth to stifle a cry.

Bite marks may be made in a variety of ways. They can result from direct pressure from the teeth, from tissue being pressed against the teeth by the tongue, or teeth scraping over tissue. These types of injury can occur singly or in combination. Bite marks are therefore often complex injuries, and their recognition and interpretation depend upon an understanding of the mechanisms involved.

Bite mark investigation starts with examination to determine if the wound can be positively identified as a bite mark. If the wound can be orientated in such a way that it is possible to say which teeth in the mouth have caused each element of the mark, then it is appropriate to make a firm statement that the wound is a bite mark. Frequently, however, an individual wound will show limited detail and it will be appropriate to identify it only as a possible bite mark.

Comparison of a bite mark with the teeth of an accused person can be achieved in several ways. The authors' preference is to detail the individual tooth features seen in the mark and those seen in the teeth of an accused. Tooth status, which describes whether each tooth has the normal size and shape for its position in the mouth or whether there is, for example, a shortened biting edge caused by a fracture, is a useful feature. Other useful features are tooth rotation and tooth displacement, where the tooth is displaced from the arch formed by adjacent teeth. Dental models of the teeth of the accused can then be compared with accurately scaled prints of the bites. Finally, the demonstration in court can be aided by superimposing transparent prints of the teeth of the accused upon the photographs of the bite mark. This is usually achieved with black and white transparent prints but occasionally, particularly in complex cases where a good visual presentation is required, superimposed colour transparencies or colour prints can be used.

Assessment of the probability of a bite having been made by a particular individual is a difficult subjective judgement requiring substantial experience and knowledge on the part of the expert. Clearly, this judgement is likely to be subjected to rigorous examination in court.

Examination and interpretation of bite marks

232 Definite bite mark. Individual marks of 19 teeth are recorded. The mark at 1 is a large mark of the upper right central incisor. Each other element can be related to an individual tooth. Each tooth has caused a tooth pressure mark where the direct application of pressure by the biting edges has caused tissue damage. There are other elements where the marks have been caused by tongue pressure pushing tissue between the necks of the teeth (arrows). Note that the bite has been photographed with a rigid scale, in the plane of the bite, close to, but not overlapping the bite.

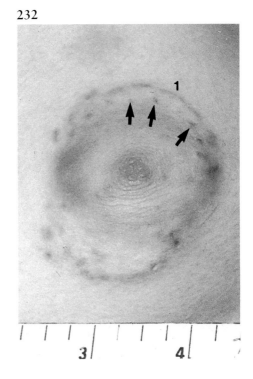

232

233 Amorous bite mark. Bites made in amorous circumstances tend to be made slowly with no movement between the teeth and the tissue. The marks adjacent to the scale were made by the lower front teeth where these were pressed into the tissue with gradually increasing pressure. The teeth are demonstrated by a red area where the tissue has been stretched over the margins of the biting edges. By contrast, the marks of the upper teeth form a series of arcs where tissue was sucked into the mouth and pressed against the backs of the teeth with the tongue. The marks represent the areas where the tissue was most stretched around the necks of the teeth and between the teeth. The area in the centre of the bite (arrows) was caused by tongue pressure pushing tissue against the rugae (ridges) on the roof of the mouth. Although this is labelled an amorous bite, the force involved is likely to have caused significant pain.

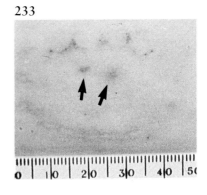

233

234 Moderately aggressive bite mark. This mark on the arm of a victim of attempted rape has been made quickly and with moderate force. The biting edges of the teeth are seen as red areas. The mark can be orientated because the two larger elements at 1 can be identified as those of upper central incisors. These two teeth marks show evidence of having scraped across the tissue before the rest of the teeth have gripped the skin to cause the main parts of the mark.

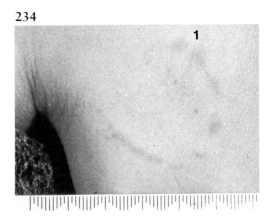

234

235

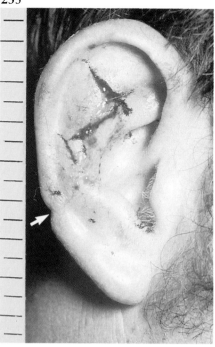

235 Aggressive bite mark. This mark has been caused by the assailant's upper front teeth pressing the ear against the side of the skull and then scraping across the tissue. This wound cannot be positively identified as a bite mark. It is not possible to say exactly which tooth has caused each element of the bite. The injury was caused by a criminal known for his tendency to bite people, and it is possible that the scar (arrow) is the result of a previous healed bite.

236

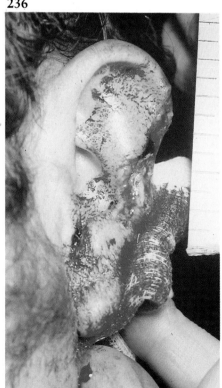

236 Very aggressive bite. The most aggressive bites can result in tissue being bitten off. This usually involves the ears, nose or nipples. Such bites can be very difficult to interpret because the tissue is usually removed by a combination of biting and tearing and it is seldom easy to relate individual parts of the mark to the individual teeth.

Variability of bite marks

It will already be clear from the preceding illustrations that bite marks can be variable injuries. In studying bite marks it is important to start with the wound, identifying the teeth which have been involved and noting any peculiarities of their size, shape or position. It is often difficult to start from an examination of teeth and predict which type of marks would be caused by individual teeth. This is because a range of factors, such as the forces involved, the anatomical site bitten and the exact biting mechanism, will vary the elements of individual teeth recorded. The variability in bites can be particularly striking in cases where multiple bites are present.

237

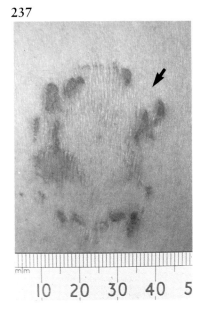

237 Aggressive bite mark. A young man was involved in an affray with four other youths. The victim claimed to have been bitten on the back. The marks nearer the ruler have been made by the lower teeth. This can be identified because the individual tooth marks are small. Several distinctive features of alignment of these teeth are evident. The marks furthest from the ruler have been caused by the upper front teeth. A gap is present (arrow), suggesting that one or more teeth is missing or perhaps much shorter than adjacent teeth and therefore has not left a mark.

238

238 Upper teeth of the accused. A bite mark in flesh is essentially a mirror-image view of the teeth. Accordingly, it is easier to compare marks with mirror-image views of the models of teeth. Shown here is the mirror-image of the model of the upper teeth of the man accused of making the bite illustrated in **237**. The features evident in the bite mark have corresponding features in the dentition of the accused.

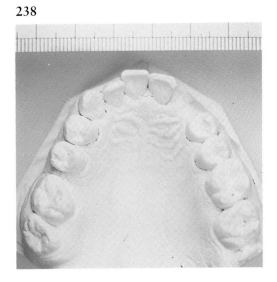

239

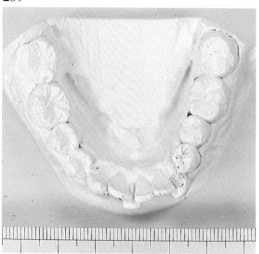

239 Lower teeth of the accused. The mirror-image view of the lower teeth shows a distinctive arrangement of the front teeth. There is marked crowding and one tooth is considerably displaced towards the lip.

240

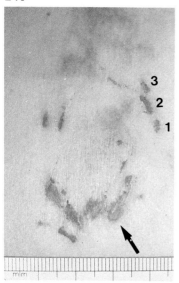

240 Second bite mark. Adjacent to the bite illustrated in **237** was another area suggestive of a bite mark. It was necessary to ascertain whether this had also been made by the accused. Initial examination suggested that these were two very different bite marks and it looked as though it would be difficult to show that this mark had been made by the same mouth as had made the mark in **237**. However, closer examination revealed that there were features of correspondence. The mark shown here had been made in a different manner, with the upper and lower teeth having made separate marks at slightly different times. The marks numbered are those of the upper left central incisor (1), upper left lateral incisor (2) and upper left canine (3). The marks adjacent to the ruler are those of the lower right first premolar (arrow) and adjacent lower right canine, lower right lateral incisor and lower right central incisor. The most prominent tooth, which was significantly longer than adjacent teeth, was the lower right lateral incisor and this is the tooth which has made two marks where it has scraped across the tissue.

Changes in bites with time

Bite marks in living victims change with time. Often, more detail is seen one or two days after the bite was made. This is probably because the initial swelling subsides allowing underlying bruising to show more clearly. There is insufficient knowledge to predict when a wound will show most detail, and it is best to photograph bites at daily intervals until there is obvious fading. In some cases variation within an individual bite occurs and detail in one area is best seen in early photographs while other areas show more detail later.

241

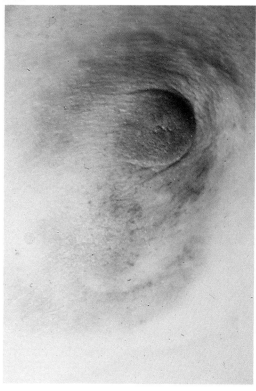

242

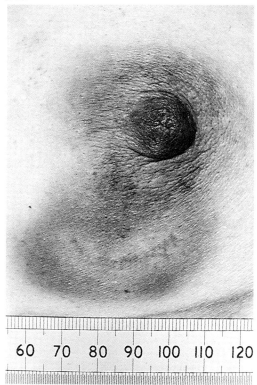

241 Bite mark, early view. This picture was obtained a few hours after the victim had been bitten on the breast. The colour photograph gives a good impression of the severity of the wound for a jury, but the detail of individual teeth is limited in this early view.

242 Bite mark, later view. The black and white photograph taken two days later shows clearer detail of the shapes, sizes and arrangement of the lower front teeth marks on the lower part of the breast. Some experts prefer to use black and white prints when making detailed photographic comparisons of the mark with transparent positive prints of the teeth of an accused person. Bite marks in dead bodies do not show the same changes with time. Occasionally they show more detail a day or so after death but there is no point in photographing them at daily intervals. However, they should be photographed before the post-mortem examination because blood is likely to drain from the bites during examination and make the marks less clear.

Bite marks in children

It has now been recognized that bite marks are an important component of non-accidental injuries to children.

243

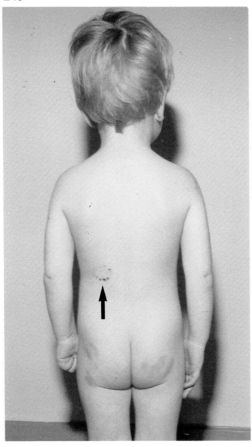

243 Bite marks on child. Bite marks are a fairly common finding in molested children. Often multiple bites are present at various stages of healing. The individual bites may show limited detail. This boy had suffered multiple bites, of which the one on the back (arrow) is the most distinct.

244

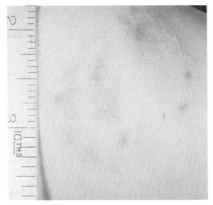

244 Detail of bite on child. This mark on the upper arm of the child shown in **243** is of the usual size and shape of a human bite but cannot be accurately orientated as there is limited detail of individual teeth. The size of the arch of teeth is evident. In this case there were five suspects. It was possible to eliminate four of these readily because their teeth could not have caused a mark of the type seen. Attention focussed on the fifth suspect and by comparing his teeth with several bites it was possible to determine that he had been the biter.

Self-inflicted bites

Where a bite mark is present on a part of the body which is accessible to the victim's mouth it is important to exclude the possibility that the bite is self-inflicted.

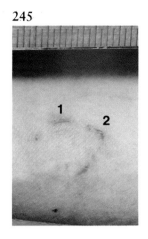

245 Self-inflicted bite. This bite was on the wrist of a prostitute who accused a young man of biting her. The mark has limited detail and cannot be orientated with certainty. The elements at 1 and 2 are towards the outer aspect of the wrist. These marks suggest the possibility of two upper central incisor teeth lying slightly at an angle to one another. The teeth of the accused man formed a broad regular arch and could not have made the bite.

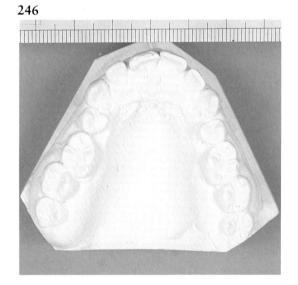

246 Victim's upper teeth. The teeth of the prostitute with the bitten wrist shown in **245** formed a relatively narrow arch with the two upper central incisors slightly angled in relation to each other. Although there was insufficient detail to be certain that the bite was caused by the woman herself, the available details all supported that possibility and when confronted with this evidence she conceded that the bite was self-inflicted.

Animal bite marks

Occasionally it is necessary to determine whether marks in flesh could have been caused by animals. This might occur when a body has been in a position where animals might have attempted to eat part of it. In such circumstances there is usually no necessity to attempt to identify exactly which animal has bitten the body. In other circumstances it may be necessary to determine whether a particular animal, such as a given dog, might have caused a bite.

247

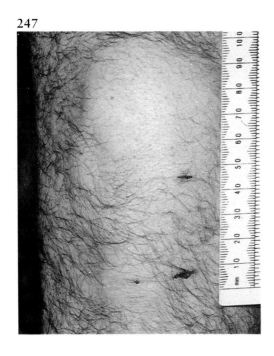

247 Dog bite mark. This bite was on the knee of a man who claimed he had been attacked by a large dog. As is usual in dog bite marks, the canine (eye) teeth have caused pointed or scrape marks, but the other shorter teeth have not reached the tissue. With such bites it is usually possible only to make an assessment of the intercanine distance, which indicates the size of the dog. In this case, the canines of the suspect dog were spaced at the same distance as shown in the bite and it was concluded that it could have made the bite.

248

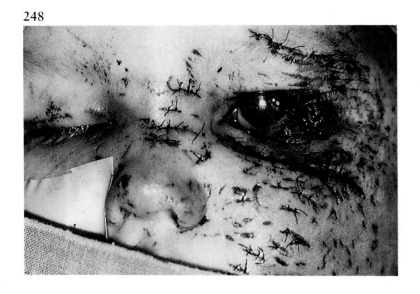

248 Rodent bites. The parents of this infant were accused of failing to protect him from an attack by a ferret kept as a domestic pet. The parents claimed that the bites were produced by rats which the local authority had failed to exterminate. The injuries can be seen to be short incised cuts and lacerations. The teeth of a ferret, which is a carnivore, would produce puncture wounds or torn flesh. These bites were made by slashes from the razor-sharp incisors of the rat.

Comparison of bite marks and the teeth of an accused person

The following series of photographs illustrates bites in a case of murder. It was possible, from examination of the marks alone to say which teeth were likely to have caused individual elements of the marks. It was possible to predict which lower teeth should have caused particular parts of the mark when tissue was bitten between upper and lower teeth.

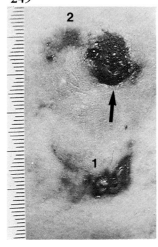

249 Bite mark on breast (actual size). The murder victim had bite marks on the breasts. The marks on the right breast are made up of two separate bites; in one the mouth is widely open and there is an arc of marks of the lower teeth (1) which was made at the same time as the mark of the upper left central incisor (2). In a separate bite the nipple (arrow) was removed.

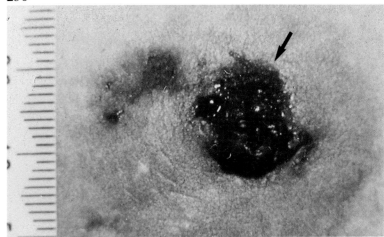

250 Detail of bitten nipple. The mark on the upper part of the bitten nipple (arrow) is a long, slightly curved mark indicative of a large tooth, the upper right central incisor. The nipple has been removed by a bite between this tooth and the lower teeth against which it bites.

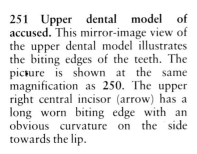

251 Upper dental model of accused. This mirror-image view of the upper dental model illustrates the biting edges of the teeth. The picture is shown at the same magnification as **250**. The upper right central incisor (arrow) has a long worn biting edge with an obvious curvature on the side towards the lip.

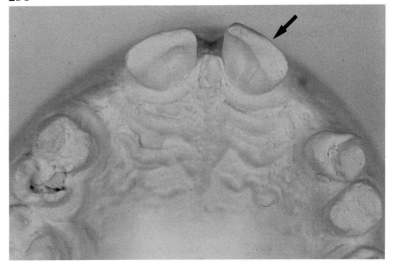

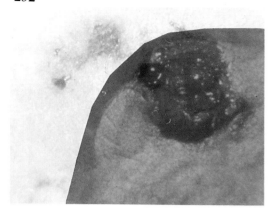

252 Superimposition of upper tooth on bite. Superimposed views of the teeth and part of the bite mark, at the same magnification, clearly demonstrate close correspondence of the size, shape and curvature of the upper right central incisor with the mark. The mark at the upper part of the area of the missing nipple could therefore have been caused by the tooth of the accused. The next question to be asked is which lower tooth or teeth would have been involved if the bite had indeed been made by the accused?

253

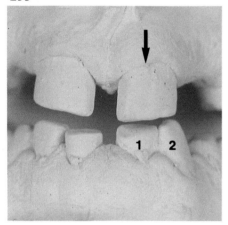

253 Upper and lower dental models. This is a mirror-image view of the upper and lower dental models of the accused as seen from the front of the mouth. The upper right central incisor (arrow) can be clearly seen to bite against two lower teeth (1 and 2). Indeed, there is obvious correspondence of the patterns of wear caused by the teeth having been ground together over a period of time.

254

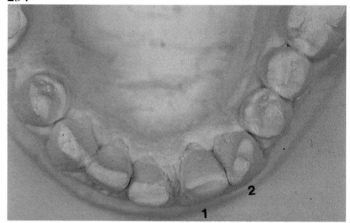

254 View of biting edges of the lower teeth. The biting edges of the lower right lateral incisor (1) and canine (2) are evident. These are the teeth which bite against the upper right central incisor. The lateral incisor has an unusual shape because the tooth has been restored by a metal-backed crown. The canine is slightly rotated. If the bite shown in **250** was made by the accused then the lowermost parts of the wound at the nipple should correspond to the teeth 1 and 2.

255

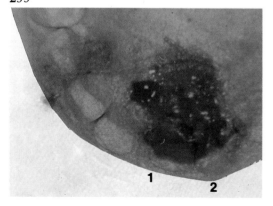

255 Superimposition of lower teeth on bite. The two teeth (1 and 2) are seen to correspond closely with the lowermost parts of the area of the bitten nipple. It can be concluded that the nipple has been removed by a bite between upper and lower teeth and the teeth of the accused show features to account for all the elements of this bite. Many other features were found to correspond between the teeth of the accused and the bites on the victim's breasts. There were no features in the bites which could not be accounted for in the teeth of the accused. The view of the dental expert expressed in court was that he had no doubt that the bite marks on the body of the murdered girl were caused by the teeth of the accused.

Comparison of the teeth of an accused with a bitten ear

In this case it was not possible to identify the mark positively as a bite mark simply by examination of the wound. However, it was possible to determine how the teeth of the accused man could have caused the bite.

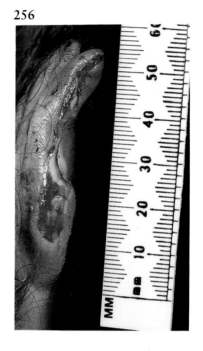

256 Bite on ear. The victim had a heated argument with his assailant, who was said to have bitten off part of the ear. Examination of the wound showed that it was of a size and shape which could have been caused by human teeth. However, it was not possible to orientate the wound in order to say which teeth would have caused individual elements of the mark. It was concluded that the wound could be classified only as a possible bite mark, and that identification of the biter from the marks on the remaining part of the ear was unlikely. The police were asked to find the part of the ear which had been removed.

257 Comparison of bitten ear with the teeth of the accused. The accused had a prominent lower jaw and could not bite his upper and lower incisor teeth together. The missing portion of ear from the wound shown in 256 could be related to the lower teeth of the accused in such a way that it was clear that the ear had been gripped by the lower canines and premolars biting against the upper teeth. The ear had then been torn off. Marks of several upper teeth were also identifiable and it was concluded that the ear had been bitten by the accused. The satisfactory outcome in this case was achieved only when the exact mechanism by which the teeth of the accused had caused the bite was determined.

257

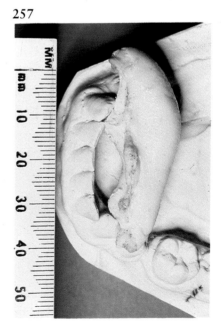

Chapter 15
Bite marks in food and miscellaneous materials

It is not uncommon for partially eaten foodstuffs to be found at the scenes of crime: much less frequently this is used for identification purposes. The foods most often found are fruits such as apples. Cheese can show excellent bite marks, but even as unlikely a material as chewing gum has been successfully used in bite mark identification.

The types of miscellaneous materials in which bite marks may be found are very varied and police officers need to have a high index of suspicion if such bites are to be recognized and used as evidence. Useful marks have been documented in materials ranging from bottle tops to wooden hairbrush handles.

The investigation of possible bites in foodstuffs and other materials is similar to that for bites in flesh. The important point is to identify the marks of individual teeth and to detail distinctive features. Corresponding features are then sought in the teeth of the accused.

If the material in which a bite is found is non-perishable it may be possible to use it in court, but in most cases photographs of the bitten material will be the best evidence. These photographs should include a rigid scale in the same plane as the bite, as for flesh marks. Bites in food should be photographed as soon as possible after being found. If this is not possible the food should be stored in a sealed polythene bag in a refrigerator until it can be photographed. Soft fruits should have a moist tissue placed over the area of the bite to stop it drying out.

It is important to recognize that bites in foods differ from flesh bites in regard to which details of the teeth are usually recorded. Marks in apples and cheese are likely to show the broadest width of a tooth where this has gouged through the material. In contrast, marks in more brittle material such as chocolate will record the indentations of the biting edges until the bitten material fractures.

Bite marks in food

258

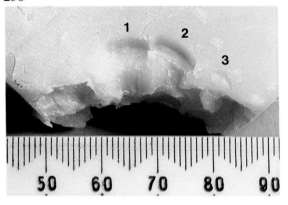

258 Cheese bite mark. This cheese was bitten and left at the scene of a shop break-in. The photograph shows the indentations of the two upper central incisors (1 and 2). The mark at 3 suggests the pointed cusp of a canine rather than the elongated edge of an incisor. The space between marks 2 and 3 is less than the width of a tooth which suggests that a tooth may be missing in this area, but that the gap has partially closed because of movement of the canine. (× 1½)

259 Cheese bite mark; photographic techniques. The detail of the photography of bite marks is very important. This is the same cheese bite as in **258**. The lighting has been altered and the tooth detail is no longer as clearly shown. It is important that whenever possible the photographs are taken under the supervision of the dental expert so that the features that will be useful in the investigation can be highlighted. The type of photographic equipment is also important. The use of 35 mm film with a ring flash is likely to produce much less satisfactory results than a larger format camera with more versatile lighting. (× 1½)

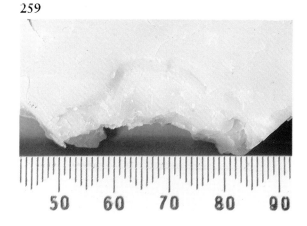

260 Cheese bite mark. The lower tooth marks in the same piece of cheese as shown in **258** show a record of the labial surfaces (towards the lip) of the teeth. These indicate where the teeth have scraped through the cheese and are likely to record marks which are broader than the individual teeth. The arrangement of the teeth relative to each other is clearly seen. The two lower central incisors (1 and 2) are in fairly good alignment. The lower right lateral incisor (3) is displaced towards the tongue and the lower left lateral incisor (4) appears to be slightly rotated with the distal part of the biting edge rotated towards the lip. (× 1½)

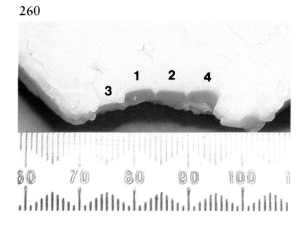

261 Bite mark in chocolate. The six lower front teeth are clearly recorded in this bite in chocolate. The nature of the marks of the front teeth varies. The canine teeth (1) show marks where the pointed parts of the teeth have penetrated into the chocolate. By contrast, the mark of the lower left central incisor (2) records the outline of the labial surface of the tooth where this has scraped through the material. Despite the varied aspects of individual teeth which are recorded, it is clear that there are distinctive features of alignment of these teeth. (× 1½)

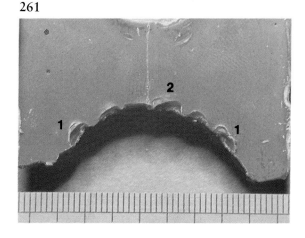

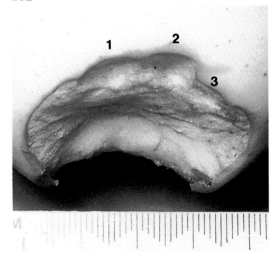

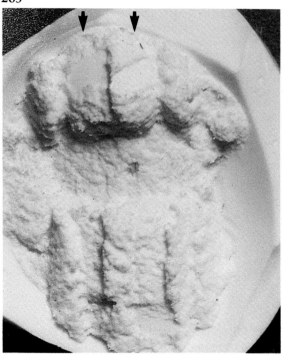

262 Bite mark in apple. Bite marks in many soft fruits are complicated by the curved nature of the bitten surface and by the fact that the material is often rotated during biting. In this bite mark on an apple found at the scene of a house-breaking the marks at 1 and 2 can be recognized as being caused by the upper left central incisor and upper right central incisor respectively. The element at 3 should be the upper right lateral incisor. The mark in the skin of the apple suggests that the tooth is displaced towards the palate. In fact this was not the case. The lateral incisor was shorter than the adjacent central incisor, and because the material had been slightly rotated during biting the lateral incisor bit into the apple later and behind the mark of the central incisor. It is important with bite marks in foodstuffs to examine the scrapes of the teeth deeper in the material. (× 1½)

263 Impression of apple bite mark. The scrape marks of the teeth through bitten material can be examined directly, but a more effective technique is to make an impression of the bitten surface with a silicone rubber base material. The illustration shows considerable detail of the labial surfaces of both upper front teeth (arrows) and the lower front teeth where these have scraped through the flesh of the apple. The upper and lower teeth have not bitten right through the material, and the 'stopping point' of the teeth can often show good detail of the alignment of the biting edges. Although it is obviously possible to make a model of the bitten apple from such impressions, it has been found more useful to use the impression as the evidence in court. (× 1½)

Bite marks in miscellaneous materials

These can be very varied, and a single unusual case is shown as an example.

264 Bite mark in tape. A rapist was in the habit of restraining his victims by binding them with the type of adhesive tape used in carpet laying. He held his victim with one arm and tore off lengths of tape with his teeth and using the other hand. Multiple marks were present on different pieces of tape. Although the series of marks illustrated shows insufficient detail to identify exactly which teeth are recorded, there is sufficient detail to allow comparison with the teeth of a suspect.

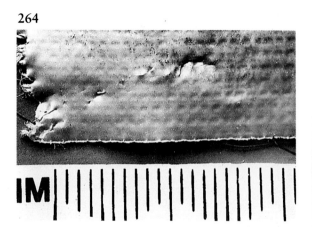

Court presentation of bite marks

Because of the varied nature of the materials bitten and the tooth detail recorded there is no single correct way of presenting such evidence in court. It is often possible to present comparisons of the bites and the teeth of an accused person in the form of direct physical fit comparisons. This series of four photographs illustrates an example in a piece of bitten cheese from the scene of a house-breaking.

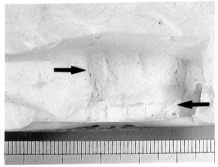

265

265 Bitten cheese. The marks of three teeth are seen in this bitten cheese. From their sizes and relative positions the marks at 1 and 2 can be identified as the upper left central incisor and upper right central incisor respectively. The mark at 3 must therefore be that of the upper right lateral incisor. These teeth are all of normal size and shape and form a regular arch.

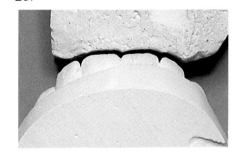

266

266 Impression of bitten cheese. The silicone rubber impression of the bitten cheese shows the shape of the labial aspects of the upper front teeth (top arrow). The biting edges of the lower teeth (lower arrow) are well shown and the arrangement of the teeth relative to each other is clear.

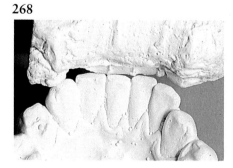

267

267 Comparison of cheese with upper teeth of the accused. In this case a model of the bitten cheese was prepared from the impressions. The cheese model and the model of the upper teeth of the accused are shown. Close correspondence of the sizes, shapes and alignment of the teeth with the marks caused by them is clearly evident.

268

268 Marks of lower teeth. The model of the lower teeth of the accused is viewed from the tongue side. The bite has been made with upper and lower teeth penetrating the cheese and then the bitten off portion being fractured away from the remainder of the cheese. The detail of the lower teeth where these have scraped into the cheese is clear and it can be seen that this corresponds closely with lower teeth of the accused. The accuracy and amount of detail evident in the comparison of the teeth and the bitten cheese allowed the expert to be confident that the bite had been made by the accused. A plea of guilty was made to the house-breaking charge.

Chapter 16
Archaeological evidence

Anthropologists and archaeologists have been quick to recognize that a multidisciplinary approach is essential if they are to interpret correctly animal or human remains found in excavations. The expertise of the dental scientist is being increasingly applied to the study of human skeletal material where the jaws and teeth are wholly or partly intact. Some archaeological investigations are restricted to a single skeleton and the investigation may proceed along similar lines to most forensic cases. On other occasions large numbers of skeletons are exhumed in the course of an excavation, and under these circumstances the situation is more analogous to the role of the forensic dentist in the mass disaster. Most of the techniques described in this book, particularly those involving the teeth and bones, may be applied in the archaeological

field, but there are certain problems which are frequently encountered in ancient skeletal material, thereby justifying their separate treatment. The examples quoted here are by no means exhaustive and most of the clinical or laboratory approaches described in other sections of the Atlas may be equally applicable in the archaeological situation.

A problem often encountered in forensic cases is how to determine whether skeletal finds are of recent origin or of archaeological significance. It may not be possible to date skeletal remains with certainty, but the colour, texture, quality and radiographic appearance of the bone may help. Fungal infiltration (see 271) usually indicates ancient origin, and the position in which the remains are discovered, for example beneath a wall of known age, can be a useful guide.

The effect of the environment

Although teeth are the most indestructible part of the human body, prolonged exposure of skeletal material to the soil may result in irreversible changes to the dentition. Because the teeth are heavily mineralized, alkaline soil conditions are most likely to result in

preservation of the teeth, whereas acidic conditions may produce considerable damage. In acid soil the enamel may be completely dissolved and excavated material would be of limited value from the forensic dentist's point of view.

269

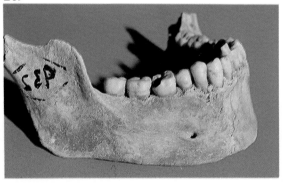

269 Well-preserved material. This mandible is from the Romano-British period dated approximately AD 400 and has survived in good condition for more than 1,500 years. Burial techniques designed to protect the body were used by some ancient civilizations, but these may result in more damage to the dental structures than when the body is allowed to decay naturally. An example was the use of gypsum by the Romano-British, the material being packed around the corpse within the coffin.

270 Partially preserved tooth. Teeth from archaeological excavations are often partially destroyed, and the cementum and dentine of the root appears to have been heavily resorbed. This resorption may have continued to such an extent that the whole of the root and coronal dentine has disappeared leaving only the enamel crown intact as a shell-like structure. Most chemicals which may be present in the soil would be expected to dissolve the enamel preferentially, leaving the coronal and root dentine at least morphologically intact. It seems likely that this tooth has been attacked by soil fungi.

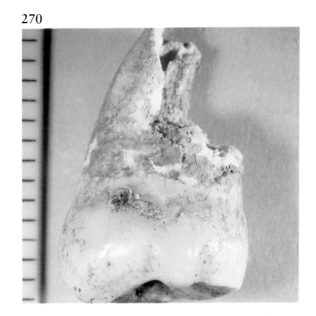

271 Fungal infiltration. This section of a tooth which had lain buried for more than 1,500 years is shown examined in polarized light. The channels produced by fungal hyphae are apparent within the dentine. The rate at which dissolution of the dentine occurs appears to be highly variable, so that some teeth, a mere 200 or 300 years of age, may show marked destruction of the dentine, whereas in other environments teeth more than 2,000 years of age may show only limited infiltration. Fungal attack does not appear to have been described in the first 50 years or so following death, so the presence of damage of this type probably indicates that the material is not of recent origin.

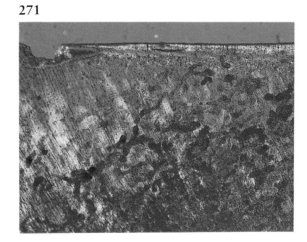

272 Tooth enamel following cremation. Although the enamel may be expected to remain intact for many centuries in non-acid environments, an exception is when bodies have been cremated. A search of the resultant fragments may produce small pieces of an almost transparent material which has been exploded off the outer surface of a tooth because of steam pressure generated within the dentine at cremation temperatures. These small fragments are often difficult to recognize as tooth enamel but may be studied by infiltration and embedding in resin followed by thin sectioning. In this example the rods or prisms of the enamel can be seen running towards the surface.

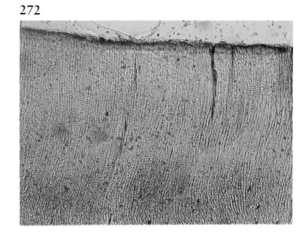

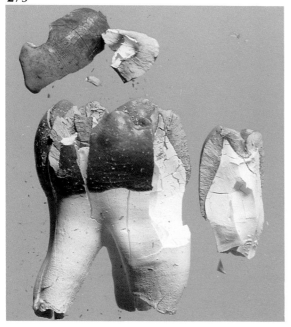

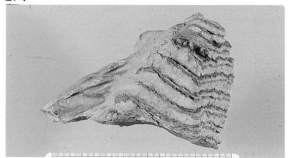

274 Fossilization of teeth. The study of changes occurring in bones and teeth after death is known as taphonomy and deals with the factors affecting the formation of fossils. Few studies have been made on human material but it is known that there are changes in the organic components in bone as well as in the crystalline structure. True fossilization is an extremely slow process and this molar tooth belonging to a mammoth and recovered from a sand pit in Southern England has been subjected to tens of thousands of years of change and is of much more interest to the palaeontologist than the forensic dentist.

275

273 Cremated whole teeth. Cremated remnants of skeletons or teeth are frequently found in archaeological excavations. As recently as 1940 it was stated that cremated remains were of no scientific interest to the archaeologist, but it would be useful at least to determine the number and type of teeth so that estimates of the size of population groups may be made. The crowns of the teeth are frequently lost as enamel splits away from the dentine. Teeth which had not been purposely dried before cremation show much less shrinkage, indicating that pre-cremation conditions may play an important part in the final result. Cremated remains are difficult to identify and forensic dentists should be aware of the possibility of error in their reports.

Teeth in antiquity

The dental and archaeological literature abounds with descriptions of the prevalence of caries in ancient civilizations. The results of such studies are of particular interest to clinical dental surgeons in that they may confirm or support current views as to the effects of diet on tooth structure, providing something is known of the diet of the early civilization being studied. Thus it has been accepted that in certain periods of our civilization the incidence of caries has been extremely low, whereas the introduction of refined carbohydrates resulted in a marked increase in prevalence.

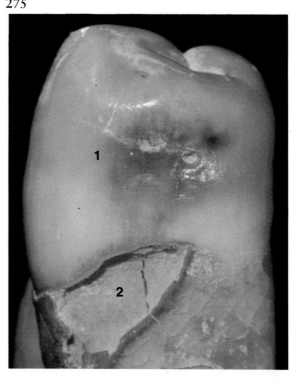

275 Caries prevalence. Studies of diets in ancient civilizations rely heavily upon determination of which teeth are carious and which are caries-free. At first sight this is a simple problem, but there may be changes in the teeth of ancient populations which have resulted from the post-mortem environment rather than from the ravages of dental decay. In this specimen of a Romano-British tooth the approximal lesion is probably caries (1) but the lesion at the gingival margin (2) could be caused by erosion from the burial environment.

276 Polarized light microscopy. Where there is doubt, specimen lesions should be prepared and viewed in the polarizing light microscope. This section is from a Romano-British tooth showing an early stage of carious attack. The lesion appears as a brown advancing front within the enamel (1), whereas the surface enamel remains intact (2). This has many of the characteristics of the modern day white spot carious lesion, and the presence of laminations within the depth of the lesion may suggest that a non-cariogenic diet has alternated with a diet of high cariogenic potential, thus resulting in some remineralization or healing of the lesion. Once a number of doubtful lesions have been checked by sectioning in this manner it is possible to arrive at suitable criteria for diagnosis of early carious lesions in an ancient population.

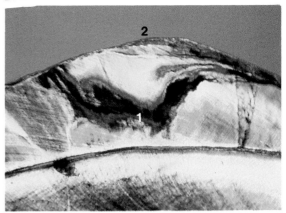

277 Untreated caries. Although primitive methods of extraction of teeth were developed in Roman times, there is no evidence that dental forceps were available in the UK until many centuries later. The ability to restore teeth to prevent the ravages of dental caries is a relatively modern development, and so it is of interest to study archaeological remains in order that the progression of non-treated dental disease can be understood. These upper premolars have suffered serious carious damage such that the crowns of the teeth have completely decayed. There is loss of bone over the apices of both these teeth and this is indicative of spread of infection to the periapical tissues. Infections of this nature in the soft tissues surrounding the mouth may have been extremely serious in the pre-antibiotic era, especially in the mandible where tracking into the region of the larynx could result in fatal laryngeal oedema.

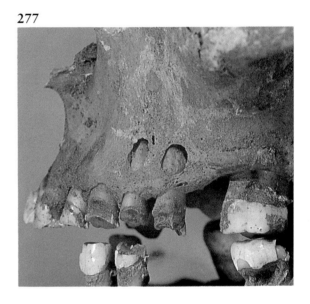

278 Attrition or wear of the teeth. This is largely caused by the abrasive quality of the diet, or of substances contained within it. The process might be expected to result eventually in an overclosing of the jaws, producing a loss of facial vertical dimension. There is evidence, however, that this does not occur and it appears that the teeth, as they become worn, continue to erupt throughout life. Wear of the occlusal surfaces of the teeth has been used in many archaeological investigations as a means of ageing individuals within the population. It has to be admitted that, at best, some of the age estimates applied to ancient skeletal material are no more than well-informed guess-work, and there is some evidence that in the older age groups the true age has been considerably underestimated.

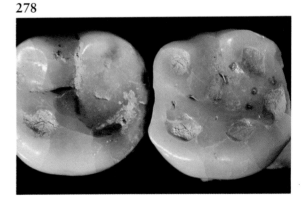

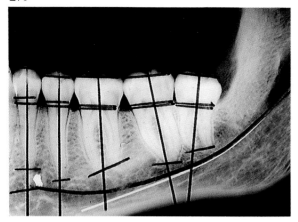

279 Continuing eruption of teeth. A useful method of collecting epidemiological data from large numbers of skeletons is by means of a standardized radiographic technique. In this case the left side of the mandible has been radiographed and distances from the upper border of the inferior alveolar canal have been measured to the apices of the teeth, to the bony margin of the alveolus, to the cervical margin of each tooth, and to the occlusal surface. Experiments of this nature have indicated that chronic infective periodontal disease is not as common as was once thought in some ancient populations.

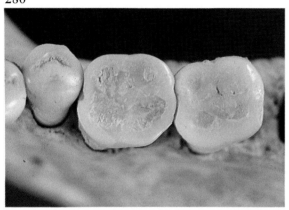

280 Approximal wear. In this example both concave and convex facetting may be seen on the surfaces of the teeth in close contact with each other. Over a lifetime a considerable amount of tooth tissue is lost during this wear process, but the teeth still remain in close contact. This is brought about by mesial drift in which the teeth tend to migrate towards the anterior part of the mouth as their approximal surfaces become worn. Very little is known about the method of formation of various facet shapes on the approximal surfaces of teeth and it is material from ancient or primitive civilizations which may help to resolve this problem.

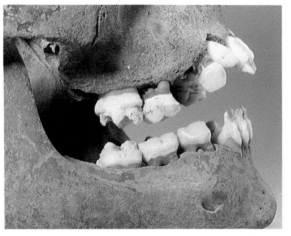

281 Developmental defects in teeth. Any interference with the normal development or structure of the enamel and dentine will produce defects which will remain more or less unaltered throughout life. The teeth are therefore particularly useful as markers of earlier disease processes. In this individual from an eighteenth century population there is severe hypoplasia of the upper and lower central and lateral incisors and of the occlusal part of the first permanent molar. Apart from contemporary records, most of our knowledge concerning diseases in antiquity is derived from studies of skeletal material and the dental pathologist has an important part to play in providing information about the lifestyle of previous populations.

The bony support

In examinations of ancient skeletal material the teeth cannot be viewed in isolation, and a study must be made of the supporting bony structures. Specimens excavated perhaps many centuries after death are rarely in perfect condition, and some teeth may have been lost entirely and not recovered at the time of excavation, or may be recovered but are separated from the jaws.

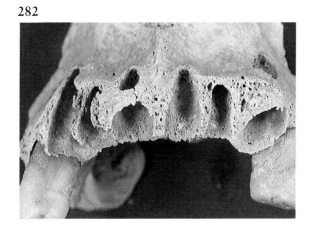

282

282 Alveolar margins. In this specimen the interproximal areas of bone have a very marked trabecular appearance, strongly suggesting that fracture has occurred after death through to the spongy part of the alveolus. From the investigator's point of view, a well-preserved sample is one in which a high proportion of teeth are either still present in the jaws or can be replaced therein, because only in these cases can adequate determination of caries prevalence be made. However, caries is, to a large extent, a symmetrical disease, so providing one half of the jaw has remained intact useful data may be obtainable.

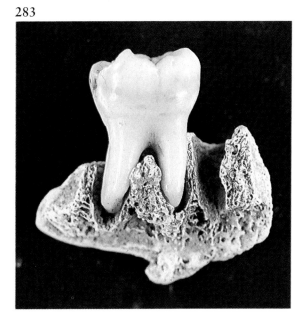

283

283 Reconstruction of fragments. The first procedure in reconstructing the dental apparatus is to identify all the teeth or fragments of teeth that have been found. Having established the identification of each loose tooth, it is common practice to replace the teeth in their original sockets. If the teeth are to be cemented in position it is preferable that this procedure be done by a dental surgeon, so that the correct occlusal relationship of the teeth be maintained.

284

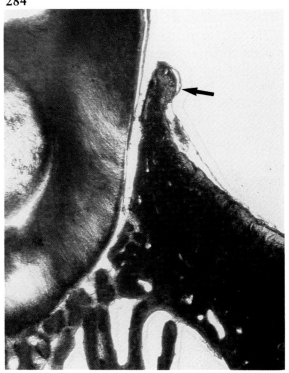

284 Reaction of bone to chronic infection. Resorption of bone is a dynamic process probably initiated by toxins and enzymes related to periodontal tissue breakdown. Bone is a living tissue capable of reacting to such an onslaught and may be capable of some repair or remodelling. It is important that the margins of the alveolar bone be examined in cases where chronic infective periodontal disease is suspected and, if necessary, ground sections taken through the alveolar margin will demonstrate reactivity in the bone. In this section through the alveolar margin of a Romano-British individual the sharp margin of the alveolar crest has been remodelled and lipping has occurred around the buccal margin of the socket (arrow).

285

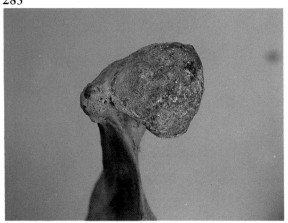

285 The mandibular condyle. This joint is unique in the body in that its movements are dependent upon and modified by the complex interdigitation of the upper and lower teeth. Loss of teeth on one side of the jaw may result in abnormal movements of the joints, whereas changes in occlusal harmony caused by attrition or caries may also be reflected in the activity of the condyles. When the joints are stressed in this way they may react by remodelling. In addition, arthritis may result in changes of shape of the condylar head, as well as in changes in surface texture. In this example there is evidence of substantial arthritic damage. Just as the forensic dentist may determine diseases present in individuals requiring identification (**96**), he or she can also advise anthropologists on diseases present in the populations they study.

286 Animal teeth and bones. Bones or fragments of bones discovered in archaeological investigations may be of animal or human origin. Dentists have a working knowledge of comparative dentitions and can distinguish between animal and human material. This skull found near human remains is that of a rat. Knowledge of animal dentitions may be needed to distinguish species, and may also be useful in a quite different context. Sometimes bones are excavated and there is clear evidence of damage by scavenging animals. Carnivores usually chew or crush bones in order to obtain the marrow and therefore will have damaged the bones in the immediate post-mortem period. Once the bones are dry they may be chewed by rodents, which produce narrow incised marks in the bone rather than crushing injuries. It may be possible to express an opinion as to the length of time for which the bones have been exposed if marks can be distinguished in this way.

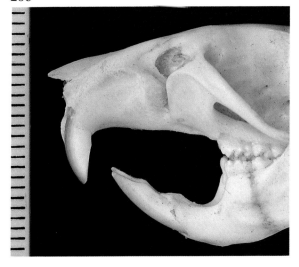

Index

References in **bold** type are to illustration numbers, those in light type are to pages.